LOW CARB
HEALTHY FAT
NUTRITION

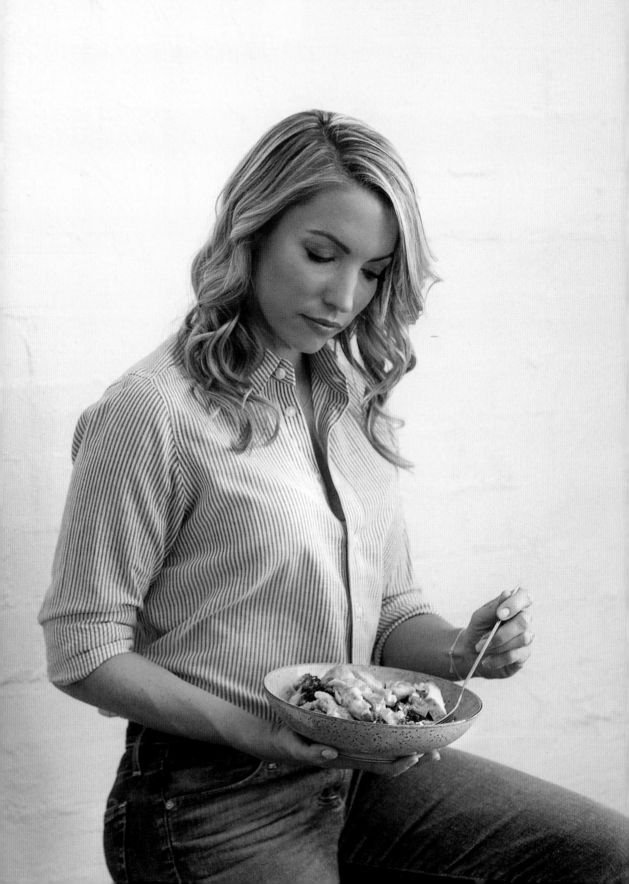

LOW CARB
HEALTHY FAT
NUTRITION

STEPH LOWE

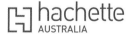

hachette
AUSTRALIA

To Ian – thank you for showing me my strength
and for always being my shining light.

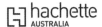

Published in Australia and New Zealand in 2018
by Hachette Australia
(an imprint of Hachette Australia Pty Limited)
Level 17, 207 Kent Street, Sydney NSW 2000
www.hachette.com.au

10 9 8 7 6 5 4 3 2 1

 A catalogue record for this
book is available from the
National Library of Australia

ISBN 978 0 7336 4014 8

Cover design by Liz Seymour
Internal design and layout by Liz Seymour, Seymour Design
Food styling and photography by Sarah Craven
Images on pages 18 and 19 by Belinda Taubman
Colour reproduction by Splitting Image
Printed in China by Toppan Leefung Printing Limited

CONTENTS

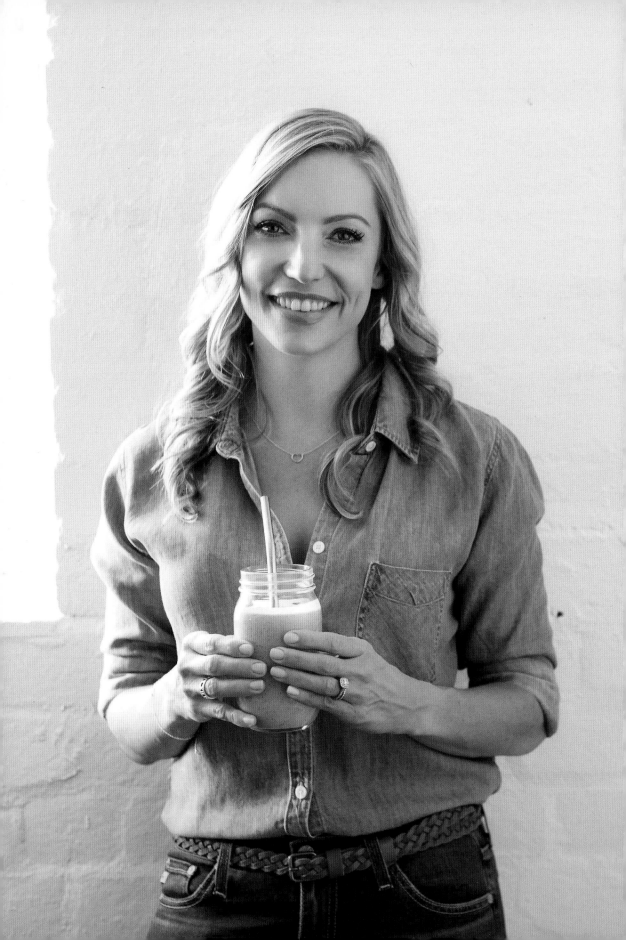

INTRODUCTION

I have been practising as a low carb healthy fat (LCHF) nutritionist since 2011 and have seen thousands of lives changed after adopting this way of life. We only need to look around our own neighbourhood to realise that chronic diseases such as obesity, diabetes, heart disease and cancer are reaching epidemic proportions, and to the science that proves how much our modern-day dietary guidelines are to blame. I am honoured to write *Low Carb Healthy Fat Nutrition* to not only present you with the research but teach you the healing power of real food.

LCHF is not a diet, it's a lifestyle. It's about reconnecting to food as it once was, before the influence of government, large-scale agriculture and 'Big Food'. It's about taking control of your health and unlocking your in-built potential to supercharge your metabolism, burn fat and extend your longevity. LCHF should first and foremost be about health, with positive flow-on effects including satiety, mood stability, appetite control, mental clarity, improved inflammatory markers and weight loss.

An LCHF lifestyle is not just about food. Together we will explore the impact of stress, but it is important that you also prioritise sleep hygiene and quality, lower your toxin exposure and include daily mindfulness for a holistic approach to health and wellness.

There are many versions of LCHF across the globe, and it is important that you use this book as a tool to find what works best for you and your health goals. My personal opinion is that LCHF should be the same as Just Eat Real Food (JERF). In terms of grams of carbohydrates per day, LCHF is a spectrum and, as we discuss, an extremely relative decision. I have chosen not to use the word 'ketogenic' in this book, as there seems to be a current division and confusion as to the exact definition of what a ketogenic diet is, and my belief is that as long as it is tailored appropriately, LCHF can be a way of life for everybody.

If you come from a low-fat background or are a serial dieter or calorie counter, please prepare to have many of your in-built beliefs blown apart. To start, all I ask for is your trust, and once you experience the benefits of LCHF first-hand, I am confident that you will never turn back. Let me hold your hand to begin this journey, but know that our bodies speak loud and clear, we just have to listen. When in doubt or when decades of knowing only one way creep back in, ask yourself, is this real food? If the answer is yes, then you are on the right path.

Real food comes out of the ground, off a tree or from an animal.

1 DIETARY GUIDELINES GONE WRONG

A LITTLE BIT OF HISTORY

To work out where we went wrong, we need to start as far back as the 1940s with the Framingham Heart Study (FHS), a long-term, ongoing cardiovascular cohort study on residents of the city of Framingham, Massachusetts.

FRAMINGHAM HEART STUDY

Under the direction of the National Heart Institute (now known as the National Heart, Lung, and Blood Institute), the FHS was a long-term study designed to identify the common contributing factors in cardiovascular disease (CVD) in a large group of participants who had not yet developed symptoms or suffered a heart attack or stroke.

Since its inception, more than 1000 medical papers have been published with reference to the study. One of the first two areas of investigation concerned how diet related to cholesterol levels and to the development of heart disease. This has led to one of the biggest criticisms and flaws of the FHS.

High dietary saturated fat levels were blamed by the FHS as a leading cause of heart disease, yet the FHS originally found that there was no relationship between fat intake and a participant's cholesterol level. The FHS also found no relationship between dietary cholesterol and serum cholesterol levels. When looking closely at the data, it can in fact be found that lowered cholesterol levels correlate with an increase of CVD death in participants over the age of fifty. At the time of conducting the research, these findings puzzled the researchers and were not included in their official report.

SEVEN COUNTRIES STUDY

We then turn to post-war Europe, when researchers in the industry noticed a decrease in the incidence of heart disease. In 1956, a researcher by the name of Ancel Keys started the world's first multi-country epidemiological study, which systematically examined the relationships between lifestyle, diet, coronary heart disease and stroke in different populations from different regions of the world.

Significantly, Keys studied the effect of dietary fat on health status. The European diet, he believed, was in vast contrast to that of Americans, who were among the best-fed individuals in the world, consuming a diet high in animal fat. Keys assumed the post-war reduction in food supply (and therefore a lower-fat diet) was a leading cause of the observed improved health status.

From 1958 to 1964, Ancel Keys's team correlated their data with heart disease outcomes in a series of regressions, plotting dietary fat intake against the heart disease deaths and assessing how closely heart disease deaths tracked with fat intake. First published in 1978, Keys's work has since come under much scrutiny. It is a well-known fact that correlation doesn't equal causation. It has also been proven that Keys selected his seven countries from ones that backed up his outcomes, when there were twenty-one for which data was available. Analysis of the full data set made the connections between fat intake and heart disease statically less clear (Yerushalmy J, Hilleboe HE, 1957). In fact, the same data set has since been used to support the positive correlation between sugar and chronic disease, but at the time this was completely ignored.

THE PLOT THICKENS – 'BIG FOOD', VESTED INTEREST AND CORPORATE LIES

In 1965 the food industry group Sugar Research Foundation paid three Harvard researchers US$6500 (approximately US$50,000 today) to single out fat and cholesterol as the dietary causes of coronary heart disease and to ignore evidence that significantly pointed to sugar as a leading cause. The 'Hegsted equation', developed by one of the researchers, Mark Hegsted, showed that cholesterol and saturated fats from sources such as eggs and meat in the diet raised harmful cholesterol levels, that monounsaturated fats had little effect and that polyunsaturated fats from sources such as nuts and seeds lowered cholesterol levels.

Published in the *New England Journal of Medicine* in 1967, their literature review, 'Dietary fats, carbohydrates and atherosclerotic vascular disease', did not disclose the Sugar Research Foundation's funding or role, but it did direct the course of our food guidelines and dietary recommendations for decades (McGandy RB et al, 1967). This paper is considered to have played the most significant role in distracting our attention away from the dangers of sugar and its role in chronic conditions including obesity and heart disease.

Unfortunately, funding from the food industry is not uncommon in scientific research. It is estimated that since 2008, Coca-Cola has spent close to $4 million on research in Australia alone and, upon analysis, their studies are five times more likely to find no link between sugary drinks and weight gain than studies whose authors reported no financial conflicts.

So, for fifty years, hundreds of millions of people were given low-fat, high-carbohydrate dietary guidelines that were arguably not supported by the evidence.

IF NOT FAT, THEN WHAT?

In contrast to Keys et al, British scientist John Yudkin was one of the pioneers in the field of research which proved the detrimental health consequences of sugar consumption. Over his career, Yudkin's research often brought him into conflict with powerful lobbies (i.e. the multimillion dollar sugar industry), but there are very few of us whose eating habits haven't been positively influenced by Yudkin in some way, whether we are aware of it or not. Yudkin's book *Pure, White and Deadly* is still extremely relevant today, over thirty years after it was written.

In 1969, George Campbell and Thomas Cleave published the paper 'Diabetes, Coronary Thrombosis and the Saccharine Disease' in the *Journal of the Royal College of General Practitioners*. They argued that chronic Western diseases such as diabetes, heart disease, obesity, peptic ulcers and appendicitis are caused by one thing: 'refined carbohydrate disease'.

One can't explore nutritional history without considering the influence of American cardiologist Robert Atkins. First published in 1972, *Dr Atkins' Diet Revolution* was one of the first low-carbohydrate diets recommended for weight loss.

Atkins was demonised by the mainstream health authorities, mostly due to the high saturated fat content of his approach, but more than forty years later it is clear how ahead of his peers he was. Revamped in 2010 as *The New Atkins for a New You*, by leading LCHF researchers Dr Eric Westman, Dr Stephen Phinney and Dr Jeff Volek, it is a *New York Times* bestseller and described as the 'ultimate diet for shedding weight and feeling great'.

REFINED CARBOHYDRATE DISEASE

Dietary guidelines in the 1970s were were largely influenced by the McGovern report, which stated, 'The diet of American people has become increasingly rich – such as meat, other sources of fat and cholesterol, and in sugar.' When we investigate the McGovern report, we discover that it was written with virtually no clinical trials to support it, and became heavily influenced by the Agriculture Committee. When asked by experts to slow down the process of writing such hefty guidelines, the researchers' response was, 'we don't have time for evidence'. On the basis of this report, the first food pyramid was developed in 1988.

Remember those three Harvard researchers paid by Sugar Research Foundation? Well, one of those, Mark Hegsted, went on to be involved in the drafting of the Dietary Goals for the United States, the predecessor of the Dietary Guidelines for Americans. In 1978, Hegsted was hired by the Department of Agriculture as Administrator of Human Nutrition and served on bodies advising the National Institutes of Health and the National Research Council in the United States, as well as the Food and Agriculture Organization and the World Health Organization internationally.

From this point in time, dietary guidelines were reviewed every five years and were continually influenced by the grain industry. It may be hard to believe that it has taken five decades for the paradigm shift we are now experiencing, but it does highlight how significantly 'Big Food', vested interest and corporate lies have influenced our dietary world as we know it. To quote Dr Eric Westman, the 'view that fat is bad in the diet has blocked the research funding into the higher fat diets'.

A PARADIGM SHIFT

Worldwide, we are now reflecting on the flawed, dogmatic and incorrect science and dietary guidelines of the past. It's time to flip the science on its head, acknowledge the mistake of decades gone and address the serious health epidemic we face – that of 'refined carbohydrate disease'. Let's take a look at what science and the leading researchers have to say.

Dr Aseem Malhotra, cardiologist and founding member of the Public Health Collaboration, has stated that dietary guidelines promoting low-fat foods were 'perhaps the biggest mistake in modern medical history, resulting in devastating consequences for public health'. Investigative journalist Nina Teicholz found, 'Saturated fat has been a healthy human staple for thousands of years, and ... the low-fat craze has resulted in excessive consumption of refined carbohydrates, which has resulted in increased inflammation and disease.'

In 2010, twenty-one past studies were included in a meta-analysis (where the results of multiple scientific studies are combined) of 347,747 individuals. The results of this study clearly state there is 'no significant evidence for concluding that dietary saturated fat is associated with an increased risk of heart disease'. So, despite five decades of low-fat propaganda, the fact is that saturated fats do not cause heart disease.

Here's what the research shows us: To put it simply, sugar consumption increases your blood triglyceride and insulin levels, which are the leading causes of chronic diseases such as coronary heart disease, type 2 diabetes, obesity and some cancers. And where does all the sugar come from? Our dietary guidelines.

The average Australian, on a Standard Australian Diet (SAD), consumes more than 40 teaspoons of sugar per day – that's without a single soft drink, item of confectionery or mouthful of junk food added. The biggest culprits are the 'healthy' foods such as low-fat yoghurt, muesli bars, cereal and fruit juice. These are, in fact, laden with hidden sugars. Worldwide, our sugar consumption has increased by 46 per cent in the last thirty years alone. Our dietary guidelines are slowly but surely killing us.

Enter: LCHF.

HIDDEN SUGARS – ON AVERAGE

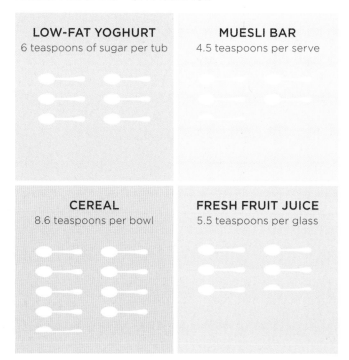

LOW-FAT YOGHURT
6 teaspoons of sugar per tub

MUESLI BAR
4.5 teaspoons per serve

CEREAL
8.6 teaspoons per bowl

FRESH FRUIT JUICE
5.5 teaspoons per glass

2 WHY LCHF?

As I mentioned in my introduction, LCHF is not a diet, it's a lifestyle. It's about reconnecting to 'real' food as it once was, unprocessed. In-built in our bodies is the ability to supercharge our metabolism, burn fat and extend our longevity. Let's take a closer look at the benefits of LCHF with a particular focus on the benefits associated with insulin, leptin and inflammation.

GLUCOSE AND INSULIN

When we consume carbohydrates, our blood glucose levels rise and the pancreas releases insulin, the hormone required to uptake the sugar into our cells. The role of the sugar is either as an immediate fuel source (glucose) or storage in the liver (glycogen). Beyond our capacity to burn or store sugar, excess is stored as fat. Many people are surprised to learn that all carbohydrates convert to sugar, even those you have been taught to believe are healthy food choices, including breads, cereal and pasta.

With excess carbohydrate consumption, especially from refined carbohydrates which are extremely poor in nutrients, our blood glucose levels resemble a roller-coaster, and the pancreas is continually instructed to release more insulin ... until the point in time when it can no longer keep up with the demands. As insulin is our fat-storage hormone, an associated symptom is significant weight gain, especially around the vicinity of the pancreas, our stomach and hips. When both blood glucose and insulin levels remain high, it is referred to as insulin resistance. When the pancreas can no longer produce insulin, the individual will be diagnosed with type 2 diabetes.

The great news is that both insulin resistance and type 2 diabetes can be avoided or put into remission by adopting an LCHF lifestyle.

Speaking of diabetes, and this may come as a shock, Alzheimer's disease is now known as type 3 diabetes, or insulin resistance in the brain. This topic deserves its own book, but the research shows that diabetics have a four-fold risk of developing Alzheimer's disease.

Leptin is our key appetite-regulating hormone, considered as the 'off switch' that stops us eating when we are full. In addition to appetite inhibition, leptin promotes thermogenesis (the metabolic process where your body burns calories to produce heat), which helps to decrease glucose and regulate body fat. With excess consumption of refined carbohydrates, however, leptin activity is blocked and your brain no longer receives the 'full' signals, so assumes it is starving – no matter how much food you continue to eat. Known as leptin resistance, it often occurs before insulin resistance but is caused by the same thing – high blood glucose levels.

The great news is that leptin loves fat, and leptin resistance can be reversed with an LCHF template. It is also important to note here that stress is another contributing factor to leptin resistance and therefore why a holistic approach is important to consider. More discussion on stress is in Chapter 10.

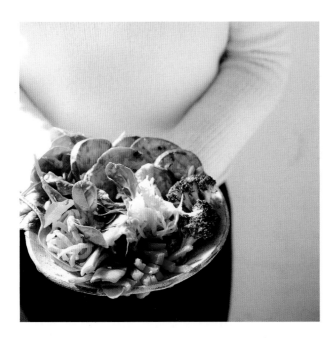

High insulin levels followed by a plummet in blood glucose causes low-grade inflammation. Glucose increases your blood triglyceride levels and starts an inflammatory cascade. Science now shows us that inflammation is the leading cause of many, if not all, diseases including coronary heart disease, type 2 diabetes, obesity and cancer. From a dietary standpoint, it is now clear that sugar is the driving factor of disease.

In summary, lowering your intake of refined carbohydrates and sugars is not just about managing your blood glucose, and burning, instead of storing, fat. It's about managing inflammation, and is essential for decreasing your risk of degenerative conditions including Alzheimer's disease, as well chronic states such as mental health conditions, cardiovascular disease and some cancers. Please share this information with your loved ones, as a properly prescribed LCHF template can slow if not reverse many chronic and degenerative conditions.

The best news: the antidote to inflammation is to Just Eat Real Food (JERF). Food that comes out of the ground, off a tree or from an animal is always the most nutrient-dense and whole-food source of nutrition. Your long-term health is in your hands and highly dependent on the food choices you make.

LCHF = JERF

When properly prescribed, a LCHF approach should be the equivalent of JERF. In addition to cutting out refined sugar, we also encourage the avoidance of the following:

- Refined seed oils included canola, sunflower and safflower oil
- Trans fats
- Poor-quality dairy
- Gluten

An anti-inflammatory approach free from the above will supercharge your metabolism and optimise your health, energy levels, hormones, performance, recovery and longevity.

3 THE SCIENCE BEHIND LCHF

Up until recently, the majority of nutrition research has been centred around conventional food guidelines, however, there are now more than eighteen randomised controlled trial studies and several meta-analyses that find improved health markers and weight control on LCHF.

Here are some of the key research papers (full citations listed on pages 244–45):

- 'Short-term effects of severe dietary carbohydrate-restriction advice in Type 2 diabetes – a randomized controlled trial' (Daly ME, 2005), in *Diabetic Medicine*, 23, 1, 15–20 – The low-carb group in this study lost more weight and had greater improvements in significant inflammatory and disease risk markers. There was no difference in triglycerides, blood pressure or HbA1c (a marker for blood glucose levels) between groups.

- 'Weight loss with a low-carbohydrate, Mediterranean or low-fat diet' (Shai I et al, 2008) – The low-carb group lost more weight than the low-fat group and had greater improvements in beneficial cholesterol levels.

- 'Carbohydrate restriction has a more favourable impact on the metabolic syndrome than a low-fat diet' (Volek JS et al, 2009) – The low-carb group lost almost twice the amount of weight as the low-fat group, despite eating the same number of calories. On the low-carb diet, beneficial changes were observed in LDL particle size, shifting to larger particles which are known to be cardio-protective.

- 'Very-low-carbohydrate ketogenic diet v. low-fat diet for long-term weight loss: A meta-analysis of randomised controlled trials' (Bueno N et al, 2013) – Individuals assigned to a very low carbohydrate ketogenic diet achieved a greater weight loss than those assigned to a low-fat diet. The study concluded that a very low carbohydrate ketogenic diet may be an alternative tool against obesity.

- 'Comparison of low- and high-carbohydrate diets for type 2 diabetes management: a randomized trial' (Tay J et al, 2015) – The low-carb diet achieved greater improvements in blood lipid profile and reductions in diabetes medication requirements, suggesting an effective strategy for the optimisation of type 2 diabetes management.

- 'Metabolic characteristics of keto-adapted ultra-endurance runners' (Volek JS et al, 2016) – Compared to highly trained ultra-endurance athletes consuming a high-carbohydrate diet, long-term keto-adaptation resulted in extraordinarily high rates of fat oxidation, whereas muscle glycogen utilisation and repletion patterns during and after a three-hour run were demonstrated to be similar.

■ 'Keto-adaptation enhances exercise performance and body composition responses to training in endurance athletes' (McSwiney FT et al, 2017) – Compared to a higher-carbohydrate comparison group, a twelve-week period of keto-adaptation and exercise training enhanced body composition, fat oxidation during exercise, and specific measures of performance relevant to competitive endurance athletes.

Future research will no doubt continue to shift away from our high-carbohydrate, low-fat message of the past and provide increased certainty as to the benefits of eating real food and turning our conventional food pyramid on its head.

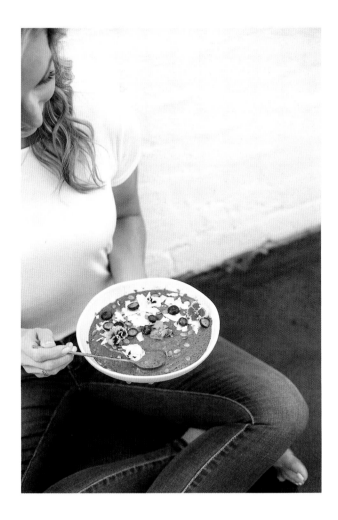

4 THE IMPORTANCE OF METABOLIC FLEXIBILITY

Metabolic flexibility is the capacity to adapt fuel oxidation to fuel availability. When you are metabolically flexible, or 'fat adapted', you can effectively burn stored fat for energy throughout the day. The term 'flexible' is used because fat burners not only have access to fat for fuel, they also have a 'dual fuel' system – they can still burn glucose when necessary and/or available, such as during high-intensity exercise. Sugar burners only have one fuel option, to burn sugar (i.e. glucose), and they can't effectively access dietary fat for energy. As a result, more fat is stored than burned.

The term 'metabolically efficient' can be used interchangeably with 'fat adapted', as fat is essentially an unlimited reserve of fuel. Even a person who weighs 60 kilograms, with 10 per cent body fat, has 6 kilograms of fat (or 6000 grams), which at 9 calories per gram is 54,000 calories to potentially access. When compared with glucose, a well-trained athlete may store 2000 calories of glucose as muscle glycogen, but this pales in comparison with having access to a dual fuel system.

FAT ADAPTATION

Fat adaptation is the metabolic reorchestration from a predominant fuel source of glucose to a predominant fuel source of fat. This is the normal, preferred metabolic state of the human. Before the modern food pyramid and dietary guidelines were imposed, humans were in a constant yearly cycle of fat adaptation, based on factors such as location, climate, season and food supply.

There are many reasons why metabolic flexibility is essential and why LCHF will not only supercharge your metabolism but support your health, performance and recovery goals, and extend your longevity. Let's take a closer look.

THE BENEFITS OF METABOLIC FLEXIBILITY

A MORE EFFICIENT METABOLISM, DAY TO DAY

With the increased ability to oxidise dietary fat for energy, you no longer need to snack every two hours. This creates a freedom from food and your appetite, it controls your energy and moods, and allows for digestive ease. Conversely, sugar burners are 'hangry' (hungry + angry) and, with the age-related decrease in glucose tolerance, often on the pathway to pre-diabetes.

GOAL WEIGHT BECOMES EASY TO MAINTAIN

As a fat burner, you can effectively access dietary fat for energy and, as a result, store less fat. Furthermore, post-prandial (after a meal) fat oxidation is increased, and again less dietary fat is stored in fat tissue. By burning fat efficiently, you can achieve your goal weight without starvation, hunger, counting calories or the metabolic disruption that comes with a calorie-restricted approach.

ENHANCED IMMUNITY

Your gut contains 80 per cent of your immune system, so it's clear that what you put in your mouth has a direct influence on your immune system. By removing refined sugar, poor-quality fats, poor-quality dairy and gluten, you are providing the essential building blocks of a healthy immune system. To this we add a gut-health practice, which you can read about in Chapter 8.

INJURY PREVENTION

Promoting an anti-inflammatory environment reduces the impact of inflammation-associated injuries. If you want to avoid this, focus on burning a clean fuel such as fat during training or racing, created predominantly by your nutrition choices meal-to-meal.

MAKING THE MOST OF MUSCLE GLYCOGEN

Carbohydrates are stored in the muscle as glycogen, but even a well-trained athlete is capped at 2000 calories. Sugar burners rely significantly on this energy source and essentially waste their glycogen on efforts that fat should be able to power. Fat burners can preserve muscle glycogen for when it is most required, such as the back end of a training session or competition, and outperform their sugar-burning counterparts any day of the week.

IMPROVED PERFORMANCE

The burning of carbohydrates results in the production of lactic acid and reactive oxygen species, which create oxidative damage that your body must mop up using antioxidants. Fats burn 'clean', however, producing only carbon dioxide and water, allowing oxidative damage to be avoided, and energy and resources to be prioritised to the recovery process. Faster recovery means you can get back out there and train better the next day, and for the entire season.

IMPROVED RECOVERY

In addition to causing constant oxidative damage when you rely on carbohydrates as a predominant fuel, processed food and refined sugars are highly inflammatory. Inflammation is extremely detrimental to your recovery and subsequent performance, so removing these foods is key.

A MORE EFFICIENT METABOLISM IN TRAINING AND RACING

When you can use fat as a predominant fuel, you direct energy outwards to working your heart, muscles and lungs, rather than inwards to digestion. Metabolic flexibility will completely change your fuelling requirements – you will no longer need 60–90 grams of carbohydrates per hour in training. You should perform consistently and finish stronger, provided your training has been optimal. You essentially become 'bonk-proof' – you avoid a 'nutritional bonk' where you run out of fuel and slow down significantly (or essentially crawl across the finish line and end up in the medical tent!)

AVOIDANCE OF GASTRO-INTESTINAL DISTRESS

Being fat adapted and no longer consuming massive amounts of carbohydrates (particularly fructose) during training and racing significantly decreases the likelihood of gastro-intestinal distress. Unlike glucose, fructose is not absorbed from the intestine but must be transported by the blood to the liver, where it is converted to glucose. It is absorbed by the intestines more slowly, which in many athletes can cause cramping and diarrhoea, especially with the high doses that are required by sugar-burning athletes.

INCREASED LONGEVITY

As sugar is highly inflammatory, a real food approach is vital if you want to prevent injuries, improve your health markers and lower your risk of chronic disease. Eating well and optimising your metabolism means you perform better, remain lean and stay metabolically healthy with age. As we have discussed, lowering your intake of refined carbohydrates and sugars is essential for decreasing your risk of degenerative conditions including Alzheimer's disease and dementia, and chronic conditions such as cardiovascular disease and some cancers.

HOW TO DEVELOP METABOLIC FLEXIBILITY

1. Lower-carbohydrate and healthier fat nutrition – This changes your physiology and allows for five or more hours between meals, based on the satiety and blood sugar response it creates. This allows for metabolic flexibility on a day-to-day basis.
2. Fasted training, or training empty – In the absence of food, fat utilisation is increased. Start with lower-intensity sessions of 1–1½ hours, and as your metabolic health improves you will find it is possible to extend this to 2–2½ hours. More than this is inadvisable in order to avoid catabolism (muscle breakdown).
3. Fasting – This topic deserves its own book, but the best way to start to strengthen your fasting muscle is by extending your overnight fast. Swapping breakfast for MCT coffee (see recipes pages 228 and 231) is a great place to start. This type of fasting is not considered therapeutic in nature but it will supercharge your metabolism and extend your fat-burning ability.

INTERMITTENT FASTING

One of the key strategies that can be used in conjunction with LCHF is an extended overnight fast, which creates a shorter eating window, known in the literature as a form of intermittent fasting (IF). We originally adopted this strategy for digestive ease and the development of metabolic flexibility and fat adaptation, but there are so many additional day-to-day and long-term benefits.

The key benefits of IF are:

- Digestive ease – as digestion is a significantly high energy-requiring process, eating less frequently can support digestive health.
- Fat loss – without the presence of circulating glucose, we increase fatty acid oxidation and can burn body fat, rather than store it.
- Development of metabolic flexibility and fat adaptation – IF is a powerful tool to becoming fat-adapted.
- Improved sleep – melatonin receptors turn off pancreas activity, so it is beneficial to eat 2–3 hours before bedtime (before melatonin is at its highest).
- Increased endurance – early research shows an increase in endurance with a 9-hour eating window, and therefore a 15-hour fast.
- Increased muscle mass development – the science is still in animal models, but restricting feeding times to a 12-hour window appears to lead to increased muscle mass, regardless of food quality.
- Breast cancer protection – a 13-hour fast in women has been shown to be protective against breast cancer.
- Chronic disease risk reduction – it lowers inflammation and the associated cardiovascular disease risk.

Intermittent fasting comes in many shapes in sizes. Some common protocols are known as the full-day fast, the alternative-day fast and the more recent 5:2 diet, which involves calorie restriction for two days a week and normal eating for five days. None of these are my preferred choice, for reasons I will discuss. My favourite protocols are as follows, conducted two days per week to begin with.

12:12 (12 hours fasting, 12 hours eating)

A 12:12 is one of the simplest strategies to optimise your metabolism (whether to become a fat-adapted athlete, to assist in fat loss or to improve cognitive function) and involves delaying breakfast. If you eat dinner late in the evening and/or eat breakfast as soon as you rise, start planning your eating times to allow for twelve hours between dinner and breakfast the next day. While it is still the most important meal of the day, breakfast definitely doesn't need to be consumed at 7am on the dot. And if you regularly eat dinner at 8pm, you will need to make portable breakfast choices to eat at your desk at 8am. With some forward thinking and simple preparation, this is easily possible.

13:11 (13 hours fasting, 11 hours eating)

A 13:11 is a great IF window and quite easily implemented as a circadian rhythm fast. Eating in line with your circadian rhythm has many benefits, including, notably, improved sleep. As we have discussed, it is ideal to eat at least two to three hours before bed, before melatonin levels peak. An example of a circadian fast will depend on what time you go to bed, but two examples are:

- Bedtime of 9pm: dinner at 6–7pm and breakfast at 7–8am
- Bedtime of 10.30pm: dinner at 7.30–8.30pm and breakfast at 8.30–9.30am

16:8 (16 hours fasting, 8 hours eating)

A 16:8 is by far the most protective fasting strategy from a disease risk point of view. Research indicates that not only does it increase breast cancer protection in women, but decreases risk factors for cardiovascular disease in both men and women. Logistically it can be more challenging, but prior planning prevents poor performance, as always. A simple example is to eat dinner by 7pm and break your fast at 11am. In women of childbearing age, I recommend the inclusion of fats in this fasting ratio, such as an MCT coffee. (This will then not be considered a therapeutic fast but will still bestow many of the day-to-day benefits we have discussed.)

Please note that it is important that you should first train your 'fasting muscle'. I do not recommend attempting a 16:8 until you have competently completed both the 13:11 and the 12:12. After you do break your fast, factors such as your ongoing satiety and exercise recovery will dictate whether you have been successful. If you fast for too long, for example, you may find that you are needing to graze following your first meal, or you may feel more fatigued in the day or days post-workout. Simply track these parameters as a way to determine when you can safely extend your overnight fast.

From an exercise standpoint, please ensure you eat within the hour after a high-intensity session. This will mean you will need to be able to finish your session fifteen hours into your fast. Aerobic training, which is (or should be) predominantly fuelled on fat, is safer to complete earlier in your fasting window, as muscle glycogen replenishment is not a primary goal at this point.

WHEN SHOULDN'T YOU FAST?

Fasting is clearly extremely beneficial for our health, but it isn't for everyone – always check with your GP first. It should definitely not be attempted under the following circumstances:

- During pregnancy or breastfeeding.
- During periods of high stress and/or adrenal dysfunction.
- If you are taking certain medications, including insulin.
- If you have poor blood glucose control. As always, start with real food first and improve your satiety and metabolism before your dive in the deep end with IF.
- After high-intensity training, as discussed.

See your Fasting Meal Plan (page 51) for more information.

5 TURNING THE FOOD PYRAMID UPSIDE DOWN

THE FAULTY FOOD PYRAMID

Our food pyramid has played a significant role in perpetuating the high-carb, low-fat message of the past. Check out the recommendations of the standard 'healthy' food pyramid: 6–11 serves of wholegrains per day; lean meats; reduced fat.

The 2017 food pyramid is a much-improved version of the original, but it still sits at 200–300 grams of carbohydrates per day, encourages the consumption of grains and tells us to minimise fat (and salt).

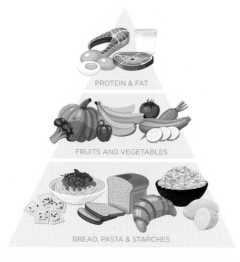

As we have discussed, carbohydrates in excess create an insulin spike, as insulin is the hormone required to uptake the sugar into your cells. If you were to follow the traditional pyramid and attempt to eat 6–11 serves of wholegrains per day, you would experience:

- Insulin spikes and crashes – the blood sugar roller-coaster
- Energy swings
- Cravings

- '3.30-itis', also known as the mid-afternoon slump
- Hanger (hunger + anger)
- A metabolism geared to sugar burning
- The requirement for 90 grams of carbohydrates per hour
- A nutritional 'bonk', where you run out of fuel before the finish line

So, in an attempt to correct the problems, you keep eating every two hours … and when traditional high-carbohydrate choices are made, a vicious cycle ensues.

Longer term, the dietary guidelines of this food pyramid can be blamed for:

- Chronically high insulin levels
- Elevated blood triglyceride
- Raised inflammatory markers
- Increased risk of chronic diseases such as coronary heart disease, type 2 diabetes, obesity and some cancers

Sound familiar? These are the same problems caused by refined sugar consumption and can be corrected with LCHF.

THE LCHF FOOD PYRAMID

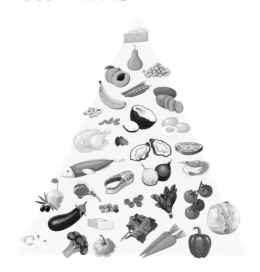

NON-STARCHY VEGETABLES

Opponents to LCHF still believe it is the modern-day Atkins Diet, when really it is an approach that celebrates plants and includes only moderate amounts of protein. The hero of the majority of your meals should be non-starchy vegetables such as spinach, broccoli, cauliflower, tomato, eggplant, mushrooms and kale. It is important to 'eat the rainbow', as the colour on your plate directly relates to its nutrient profile.

The health benefits of non-starchy vegetables include:

- Rich in vitamins A, C and K
- High in antioxidants and extremely anti-inflammatory
- High in phytochemicals and polyphenols
- Natural fibre and therefore digestive support

HEALTHY FATS

As you are now well aware, when it comes to current dietary guidelines, the demonisation of fat still exists. Fat will make you fat? WRONG; fat will help you *burn* fat. Remember this mantra when old habits creep in, or naysayers get in your ear: good-quality fats provide nutrient density, satiety, hormonal control and an anti-inflammatory approach.

Our two key groups of healthy fats are:

1. Omega-3s

These are our anti-inflammatory fats, (not to be confused with inflammatory omega-6s such as refined seed and vegetable oils). Examples include avocado, nuts, seeds, olives, olive oil and grass-fed animal products. The health benefits of omega-3s include:

- Fat-soluble vitamins A, D, E and K
- Improved memory and cognition
- Increased skin integrity
- Decreased inflammation

2. Saturated fats

Saturated fats include coconut oil, butter, ghee, MCT oil, animal fat and full-fat dairy (if tolerated). Their health benefits include:

- Providing the building blocks for our cell membranes and hormones
- Acting as carriers for our important fat-soluble vitamins
- Providing a concentrated source of energy to steady blood sugar and insulin
- Turning you into a fat-burning machine!

QUALITY PROTEINS

Examples of quality proteins include eggs, fish, chicken, turkey, beef, lamb, kangaroo, tofu and tempeh. When it comes to animal products, it is extremely important to consider quality, as 'you are what you eat eats'. Knowing whether your animal products are pasture raised, free range and grass fed are important purchasing decisions from both environmental and health perspectives. The environment that an animal is kept in and the quality of the food provided directly affects the meat and egg quality you consume. Please avoid grain-fed protein, as this promotes a high omega-6 and therefore inflammatory environment. The health benefits of quality proteins include:

- Blood sugar and craving control
- Cognitive function
- Lean muscle mass development
- Neurotransmitter production, and therefore mood balance
- Body fat reduction

What about 'organic?'

By definition, certified organic produce comes from animals kept on farms which meet and exceed standards of the best free-range facilities. The problem is, however, that the word 'organic' may merely mean that animals in barns are fed organic grains. It does not mean the welfare of the animals meets certified standards. There can certainly be health benefits of consuming organic produce, but it is safest to prioritise organic only when you can ensure the animal is also pasture raised, free range and grass fed.

WHOLEFOOD CARBOHYDRATES

It is important to understand that non-starchy vegetables are by definition wholefood carbohydrates, but per gram they are much lower in carbohydrate than starchy carbohydrates in this category. With LCHF, wholefood carbohydrates are best added post high-intensity training. We discuss the amount you require in Chapter 10. The best sources of wholefood carbohydrates are fruits such as bananas, apples and oranges, starchy vegetables such as sweet potato, potato and beetroot; and gluten-free grains such as basmati rice, buckwheat and quinoa. The benefits of wholefood carbohydrates include:

- Natural fibre and therefore digestive support
- Fuel for glycolytic activity (e.g. high-intensity exercise)
- Muscle glycogen replenishment
- High levels of tryptophan, and therefore relaxation and improved sleep
- Resistant starch for a healthy gut microbiome

6 HOW TO BUILD YOUR PLATE

We have provided you with an abundance of meal plans and recipes, but it is important to arm yourself with the skills to build your plate effectively. This not only ensures nutrient balance and satiety, but it allows you to learn how to compose simple meals for when you're time-poor and to make the best choices from café or take-away menus.

BUILD YOUR PLATE – Females 2:1:1 or 2:1:2 (relative to meal frequency)

1. Consume two (2) cups of predominantly non-starchy vegetables at every meal.

2. Consume one (1) serve of protein at every meal.

3. Consume one (1) to two (2) serves of good fats at every meal.

4. Complex carbohydrates are optional and, if required, should be added to your plate last, and predominantly post high-intensity training (PT). Please start with ½ cup and increase if necessary. This decision should be made on factors such as ongoing satiety, and training performance and recovery.*

BUILD YOUR PLATE – Males 2:1:2

1. Consume two (2) cups of predominantly non-starchy vegetables at every meal.

2. Consume one (1) serve of protein at every meal.

3. Consume two (2) serves of good fats at every meal.

4. Complex carbohydrates are optional and, if required, should be added to your plate last, and predominantly post high-intensity training (PT). Please start with 1 cup and increase if necessary. This decision should be made on factors such as ongoing satiety, and training performance and recovery.*

* A note for endurance athletes: If you are heading out for a long fasted session the next morning, a portion of complex carbohydrate included with your meal the night before can be beneficial (the caveat to our nutrient-timing principles). Once you have trialled this, it may be incorporated as potential race-day strategy. A simple example is the addition of sweet potato to your Friday-night steak and salad.

BUILD YOUR PLATE EXAMPLES

Building your plate is as simple as JERF – that is, choosing food that is whole and unprocessed. Some examples include:

1   A three- or four-egg omelette with spinach, tomato and mushroom, served with half an avocado.
2   A smoothie including avocado, coconut cream, protein powder and spinach. After high-intensity training, add 1 banana.
3   A salad of spinach, tomato, capsicum, walnuts and tuna, topped with an olive oil and apple cider vinegar dressing.
4   A salmon fillet served with steamed greens topped with grass-fed butter and sea salt. After high-intensity training, add ½–1 cup sweet potato mash.

MACRONUTRIENT SERVING SIZES (1 serve equivalent)

NON-STARCHY VEGETABLES (~2 cups / meal)

asparagus	alfalfa	spinach	cucumber
leek	zucchini	lettuce	pumpkin
onion	celery	kale	cabbage
broccoli	cauliflower	capsicum	tomato
Brussels sprouts	bok choy	mushrooms	carrots

Please note: This list is not exhaustive. For the purposes of our version of LCHF, any green vegetable is considered non-starchy. Please minimise corn, as it is a grain.

PROTEIN (~1 serve / meal)

1 palm-size piece of fish, chicken, beef, lamb, tofu or tempeh
    (organic and non-GMO) (F – 120g; M – 150g)
1 can tuna, salmon or sardines (F – 90g; M – 180g)
3 free range eggs OR 2 eggs + 50g bacon OR 2 eggs + 30g cheese (F)
4 free range eggs OR 3 eggs + 50g bacon OR 3 eggs + 30g cheese (M)
30g (F) or 45g (M) protein powder
1 cup lentils, legumes and/or chickpeas
3 tablespoons hemp seeds + ½ cup lentils, legumes and/or chickpeas
    (please count hemp seeds as 1½ serves of fat)

FATS (1–2 serves / meal)

½ large avocado

30g grass-fed butter or ghee

30g nuts or seeds (limit cashews due to high carbohydrate
content; peanuts are legumes)

30ml flaxseed, coconut, macadamia, hemp, avocado or extra-virgin
olive oil

15ml any of the above oil + 1 tablespoon nuts or seeds

½ cup coconut cream or milk (BPA-free can)

Please note: One (1) serve of most animal proteins (exceptions are chicken breast,
tuna in spring water, etc) and one (1) serve of free range eggs provide approximately
½ a serve of good fats. For your main meals it is likely you will need to add ½ a serve
to create 2:1:1 and 1½ serves to create 2:1:2.

COMPLEX CARBOHYDRATES (BEST CONSUMED PT)

1 piece (F) or 2 pieces (M) fruit (e.g. banana, apple, orange)

½ cup (F) or 1 cup (M) starchy vegetables (e.g. sweet potato,
potato, beetroot)

½ cup (F) or 1 cup (M) basmati rice, buckwheat or quinoa (cooked)

1 slice (F) or 2 slices (M) gluten-free bread*

* Please note: Bread is obviously not JERF, but if you choose to eat it occasionally
then it forms a part of the balanced approach we are striving for. Where possible,
ensure quality by making a selection from your local health-food store.

7 STARTING LCHF – THE METABOLIC GREY ZONE

If you are a complete sugar burner due to previously high carbohydrate consumption, the first three to four days on LCHF can be challenging. Known as the 'metabolic grey zone', it is a period in which the body has an inability to burn fat, even though relatively few carbohydrates are being consumed. During this time, the overall energy provision feels low, even in the case of higher-than-normal calories. Initially this can contribute to fatigue, hunger, headaches, low moods and poor performance. It is important to understand this transition and know that if you stick to your LCHF template it will be over in a matter of days. As your metabolic flexibility improves and your body learns to burn fat, your symptoms will disappear.

To assist your transition, the following can help:

1. If you are used to consuming high volumes of refined sugar and/or caffeine, gradually reduce your intake in the weeks prior to starting LCHF. Many of the aforementioned symptoms are caused by the detoxification process that takes place when you decrease your reliance on these 'drug-like foods'.
2. Stay hydrated. It may sound overly simple, but thirst is often mistaken for hunger. Make sure you are consuming at least 2 litres of water per day, and add fresh lemon and rock salt for natural electrolytes.
3. The fear that salt with give you high blood pressure and kill you is another dogma-based myth of the last five decades. As you become fat-adapted, your salt requirements increase dramatically, so please add salt liberally to your meals to maintain optimum blood volume. If you experience fatigue or poor performance beyond the metabolic grey zone, it is essential that you experiment with a higher salt intake before assuming that any additional carbohydrates are required.
4. Work on your fat phobia. Our calorie-counting and low-fat ways of the past can trip you up. You are now free to eat butter, avocado and full-fat foods, but you may have a strong in-built fear of these foods. You simply cannot cut carbohydrates and fat at the same time. If you're hungry within five hours of eating, add more non–starchy vegetables and good fats and watch your satiety extend.

5. Rest. It's important to listen to your body during this time. If you need to take a day or two off training and have an early night, then please do. Adequate rest and quality sleep are just as important as the food choices you make.

After this initial phase, there are so many benefits. The biggest difference experienced day to day is satiety, shifting from insatiable hunger and snacking every two hours, to being well-fuelled for five or more hours in between meals. The case of hanger (hunger + anger) is a thing of the past, and it is quite life-changing for most. And it's this satiety that keeps the benefits continuing – as we have discussed, when you don't need to eat for five hours, you open up a huge fat-burning opportunity between meals.

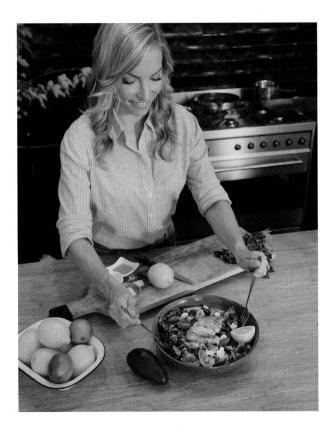

8 THE IMPORTANCE OF GUT HEALTH

Gut health is the cornerstone of your health and immunity. Here is some food for thought (pun intended!):

- Your gut really is your second brain, with more than 95 per cent of serotonin receptors located there.
- There are approximately 3 kilograms of bacteria in the gut – that's more bacterial cells than human cells. Did you know that we are actually 90 per cent bacteria? Kind of gross, but mind-blowing nonetheless!
- Your gut and brain are connected via your vagus nerve, and addressing this connection is often a key missing element in the treatment of:
  - mental health conditions such as anxiety and depression
  - digestive disorders including small intestinal bacterial overgrowth irritable bowel syndrome and irritable bowel disease
  - autoimmune diseases such as multiple sclerosis, rheumatoid arthritis and Hashimoto's disease

WHY IS GUT HEALTH SO IMPORTANT?

Gut bacteria assist in food breakdown, help produce essential nutrients and allow for greater nutrient bioavailability (via pre-digestion). Without the right balance, nutrient production, absorption, digestion and assimilation is sub-optimal. This has powerful implications for: health and vitality; immunity and protection from food allergies and intolerances; cognition, memory and overall brain health; natural detoxification pathways; growth in children and adolescents; exercise performance and recovery; weight loss ability; and the list goes on ...

WHY IS MY GUT HEALTH NOT SELF-REGULATED?

There are many reasons why we now realise that the world we live in, our choices and our behaviours are no longer supporting our gut health. Here are just a few:

POOR NUTRITION

Prior to the recent real food revolution, refined sugars, refined seed oils, trans fats and gluten were everywhere. These inflammatory foods kill good gut bacteria and allow bad bacteria to thrive. Our ancestors didn't eat anything in a box, so why should we? Not to mention that our ancestors also had to ferment (i.e. preserve) their foods, as they had little other choice. With the introduction of refrigerators, canning and preservatives, the probiotic nature of traditional foods has been destroyed.

STRESS

Living in today's Western society, we are stressed, busy and chronically tired, and with our constant exposure to heavy metals and environmental toxins, our gut just sometimes can't stay healthy. Stress is significantly detrimental to gut health, and while it can't be completely avoided in the modern world, stress management techniques such as meditation and mindfulness, and minimising your toxin exposure (such as those found in conventional cleaning and beauty products), are important in promoting gut health.

MODERN MEDICINE

Antibiotics, synthetic prescriptive drugs, the oral contraceptive pill ... Did you know that your gut health is passed down from your mother at conception? If your mother was ever on the contraceptive pill, it is highly likely that your gut health has been disrupted. The pill acts like antibiotics and kills off the beneficial bacteria in the gut. If you are still taking the pill yourself, it is time to learn another way of contraception. If you are taking the contraceptive pill to address an underlying issue, such as acne or painful periods, it is time to get to the root cause of the problem rather than putting a band-aid over the top.

HOW DO I KNOW IF MY GUT HEALTH IS SUB-OPTIMAL?

Honestly, you'll know. As Hippocrates said, 'All disease starts in the gut.' So too does all health. Burping, flatulence, bloating and excessive noises coming from your stomach are not normal. If you are experiencing any of those symptoms, or unusual cravings, poor bowel movements or unexplained headaches, start healing your gut today.

It's not just the more obvious digestive symptoms, though. Acne, eczema, skin rashes, pre-menstrual syndrome, fatigue and unexplained headaches all have roots in poor gut health.

Remember we also discussed glucose, inflammation and your brain? Research into mental health conditions including depression and anxiety is strongly linked back to our food choices and the state of our gut health, or internal ecosystem. Many people worldwide who are now switching to a LCHF lifestyle with a gut-health focus are, over time, reducing or even removing their need for pharmaceutical intervention. Amazing, isn't it?! (Please note: the operative words are 'over time'. I am not suggesting you change any of your current medications and, as always, please discuss this with your GP before making any adjustments.)

WHERE DO I START?

The best place to start is where you are comfortable, and below are a number of options to begin your gut-health journey. Please note, it is not a matter of 'more is more', as you can overdo even the good bacteria. Please start gradually and build your intake over the next four weeks.

FERMENTED VEGETABLES

Fermented vegetables are one of the easiest and most convenient sources of good bacteria. Fermented foods in general contain millions of beneficial microbes, which drive out pathogens and therefore protect gut integrity. In addition, the bacteria pre-digest our food, which means we have greater access to nutrients. There is actually twenty times more bioavailable vitamin C in sauerkraut than in fresh cabbage.

Fermented vegetables are also the most economical place to start – see the recipe for sauerkraut below. If you prefer to purchase your fermented vegetables, they are available in the fridge section of most health-food stores.

MAKE YOUR OWN SAUERKRAUT

To make sauerkraut, finely shred a cabbage and place in a large bowl. Stir in a tablespoon of rock salt then use your hands to squeeze as much juice out of the cabbage as possible. Retain the juice and transfer both it and the cabbage to an airtight container. For large cabbages, you may like to split this process into two batches. Salt is essential to create the right environment (pH) for fermentation to take place.

Once all the cabbage is well packed into the container and covered in juice, all you need to do is seal it tightly and store it on the kitchen bench for 4–7 days. Then transfer to the fridge, and enjoy as required. Try serving 1–2 tablespoons on your eggs, in a salad or as a side to any main meal.

TIP: You can use any vegetables you like (for example, carrots, beetroot, daikon and artichokes), in any combination, and add any herbs and spices you desire.

BONE BROTH

Bone broth is one of nature's true superfoods. It is packed full of calcium, magnesium and phosphorus, and provides gelatin and collagen for cell integrity and healing. While everyone will benefit from consuming bone broth, it is absolutely essential for those with leaky gut, celiac disease, Hashimoto's disease and other autoimmune conditions.

This mineral-rich drink or stock is also one of the best ways to ensure your kitchen is wastage free. Our Super-easy Bone Broth recipe is a great place to start (see www.thenaturalnutritionist.com.au). If you are not quite ready to make your own, you can buy dehydrated bone broth products online and rehydrate as required.

YOGHURT

A probiotic yoghurt is one of the simplest ways to consume fermented foods regularly. Making your own with a starter culture is highly recommended – in fact, it's so beneficial that it needs to become your predominant gut-health food. Here's why:

- It is fermentation made easy. All you need to do is purchase your starter culture and add it to coconut cream to make yoghurt, or coconut water to make kefir. It requires only a small investment of your time, and no elaborate equipment. Dairy-free options are preferable but you can consider milk-based yoghurt or kefir if tolerated.
- The starters contain multiple strains of good bacteria, which is important for microbiome diversity. Many commercial probiotics contain only two strains.
- One starter can be used to make approximately 10 litres of yoghurt. It then works out as only a few dollars per litre – one of the most cost-effective ways to prioritise your gut health.

KEFIR

Kefir is a probiotic drink made from 'grains' (tibicos) which act like the starter culture in yoghurt. Traditionally, the grains are added to milk and fermented via the lactose, or milk sugar. Dairy-free and vegan options are also available. Similar to yoghurt, it is as simple as combining the starter with coconut water in a glass jar, sealing and fermenting on the bench for 4–7 days.

If you're not quite ready to DIY, there are some dairy-free, sugar-free and delicious yoghurts and kefirs available in health-food stores.

KOMBUCHA

Kombucha is made from a starter culture (symbiotic colony of bacteria and yeast, or SCOBY), sugar and tea. When double fermented, it becomes a fruity fizzy drink and a great replacement for soft drink.

To make your own, obtain a SCOBY from someone already brewing their own kombucha tea, purchase one from a reputable source, or grow one from a bottle of raw (i.e. unpasteurised) kombucha tea. I prefer the latter, and my how-to instructions are online at www. thenaturalnutritionist.com.au

THE IMPORTANCE OF RESISTANT STARCH

By now you are aware of the benefits that probiotics have on our health, and in particular our gut health. But have you ever considered the importance of *prebiotics* in the human diet? One form of prebiotic that is often overlooked is resistant starch. Resistant starch is a type of food starch that remains intact through the stomach and small intestine, reaching the large intestine (colon) in its whole form. So as the name suggests, resistant starch is resistant to digestion by the host.

When resistant starch reaches the large intestine it begins to ferment, and colonic bacteria break it down into short-chain fatty acids. These fatty acids are the main source of nutrition for the friendly bacteria in the gut and therefore promote healthy gastro-intestinal function, improve gut mobility and decrease the risk of leaky gut and inflammatory conditions of the bowel. Due to the indigestible nature of resistant starch, it can also improve insulin sensitivity and lower blood glucose levels, and it has close to no calories.

Like any other organisms, bacteria found in the gut require nourishment, and certain food types are more superior than others. Resistant starch is the highest-quality food for your gut bugs, however consideration must be made when choosing food sources.

TYPES OF RESISTANT STARCH

There are four types of resistant starch, some good and some not so good:

1. Starch bound within cell walls, found in grains, seeds and legumes. Some of these foods can cause digestive issues in many individuals due to processing methods and the gluten content, therefore this type of resistant starch is not ideal for everyone.
2. Intrinsically indigestible starch (due to high amylose content), found in foods such as green (unripe) bananas and raw white potatoes. This type can also be found in a powder form, such as green banana starch or unrefined potato starch. This is a great option – just make sure you opt for unrefined and natural powders that are made with no other added ingredients.
3. Starch formed after one of the above starches has been cooked and rapidly cooled, such as cooked and cooled white potato, sweet potato or white rice. This is a cost-effective method of consumption and a great

way to begin testing out resistant starch. It is my preferred way of ensuring that LCHF does provide adequate food for your beneficial gut bugs to thrive.

4. Industrial starch that has been chemically modified and should be avoided at all times.

That being said, I am not advocating a bowl of potato salad or carbohydrates that have been cooked and cooled every day, and consideration must be made when adding resistant starch into your diet, as it can be quite a balancing act. Start with very minimal amounts, for example half a teaspoon in powder form and increase as tolerated, aiming for 1 or 2 tablespoons per day. This is to avoid symptoms such as bloating or gas, which can often be a side effect if not consumed correctly.

9 THE CALORIE FALLACY

One of the biggest myths of the last five decades is what we refer to at The Natural Nutritionist as 'The Calorie Fallacy'. For fifty years we have been told that weight gain or weight loss is a measure of energy in versus energy out, and therefore that to lose weight you must simply be in calorie deficit. Through the 1970s and 1980s this led to an abundance of calorie-counting diets, the appearance of weight-management companies, 'low-fat', 'lite' or non-fat 'food-like' products, and the popularity of slogging yourself at the gym to burn thousands of calories.

It is important to understand that physiology is not maths, nor physics for that matter. The point of this chapter is not to debate the first law of thermodynamics (which, by the way, refers to a closed system and is utterly irrelevant), but to share with you some great news – it's not about eating less and exercising more, it's about real food. Here's why:

1. CALORIES ARE NOT CREATED EQUAL

Our macronutrients (i.e. carbohydrates, proteins and fats) produce varying hormonal responses and therefore metabolic environments, which either promote or discourage fat storage.

- Example A: Carbohydrates are equivalent to protein in energy, but when eaten in excess can lead to chronically elevated insulin levels. This is the recipe for fat storage. Long term this will create insulin resistance, the precursor to obesity and diabetes.
- Example B: Fats are more than double the energy of carbohydrates and protein, but offer satiety and hormonal control – the keys to long-term fat loss. Healthy fats exclude refined seed or vegetable oils and trans fats, of course. On that note, low-fat food products belong in the bin. They are not whole foods, and most of the time they are higher in sugar than the full-fat version. See Example A.

2. FAT LOSS IS ABOUT HORMONAL CONTROL

Hormonal control comes not only from managing your carbohydrate intake (to control insulin) but also from controlling your stress. With efficient stress-management techniques, you manage the stress hormone cortisol and continue to promote a fat-burning environment. Eating less and exercising more are huge stressors for the body, and ironically can lead to weight gain, often seen as the 'cortisol pouch' – that stubborn abdominal fat around your middle.

3. THE THERMIC EFFECT OF FOOD

The amount of energy required to break down our macronutrients – known as the thermic effect of food – varies significantly. Your body burns far more calories digesting protein and fibrous vegetables than it does simple sugars like pasta, white bread or packaged cereals. Digestion actually requires a large amount of energy (this is a good thing!), which can be accelerated with better food choices. You can truly turn your body into a fat-burning machine.

4. FOOD QUALITY CREATES NATURAL PORTION CONTROL

If you focus on food quality, the quantity will take care of itself. After all, it's very uncommon to gorge oneself on broccoli or binge on chicken. Fill your plate with predominantly non-starchy vegetables, quality protein and good fats from salmon, avocado, grass-fed butter, coconut oil, nuts and seeds, and you will be so satisfied that you won't go near the bread basket or even consider that lemon meringue.

Please note: It's not about gluttony, but 800–1200 calories is the recipe for metabolic dysfunction, where your metabolism slows and eventually your body goes into starvation mode. Starvation is not healthy. The answer is to nourish your body with food as nature intended.

10 THE CARBOHYDRATE FALLACY

When you manage your carbohydrate intake (hormone: insulin) and your stress (hormone: cortisol), your insulin remains low, which keeps you in our preferred metabolic state of fat burning. Remember:

Low Insulin = Fat Burning

SO HOW MUCH SHOULD I EAT?

We have also discussed how carbohydrates in excess create an insulin spike, as insulin is the hormone required to uptake the sugar into the cells. So it's about finding the sweet spot – adequate consumption (because we know how important fruit and vegetables are) without excess insulin.

How much?

The answer is, it depends. For example:

- A 'metabolically healthy' endurance athlete might need 150 grams of carbohydrates per day.
- A sedentary person will most likely need less than 100 grams of carbohydrates per day.
- Type 2 diabetics often need less than 25 grams of carbohydrates per day, at least in the initial stages.

To further define your current level of metabolic health and individualise your daily carbohydrate requirements, there are three main fasting blood tests your GP can run. These are:

1 Blood glucose level: ideal ~5.0 mmol/L
2 Fasting insulin: ideal 3.0–5.0 mIU/L
3 Glycated haemaglobin – HbA1C (%): ideal <5.3%

The higher your levels, the more carbohydrate resistant you are and the less you should consume. HbA1C in particular is one of the most important blood tests in medicine. It measures the three-month trend of the sugar stuck to your red blood cells and indicates whether you are metabolically healthy, or moving towards a pre-diabetic or diabetic state. If you have a HbA1C >5.3%, you will need to lower your carbohydrate intake closer to 50 grams per day, relative to your activity levels. A HbA1C of 6.5% is the criterion for diagnosing diabetes, and carbohydrate levels must be lowered further to avoid pharmaceutical intervention. As you now know, LCHF is a powerful strategy to reverse type 2 diabetes, and you can learn more in our 14-Day Diabetes Management Plan on page 49.

A NOTE ON STRESS

In situations of stress, our adrenal glands produce the hormone cortisol. This is part of our 'flight or fight' response and is necessary to human optimal function and survival.

The role of cortisol is to stimulate the liver to release glucose into the blood, so that in caveman days we were supplied with an immediate source of fuel in order to run away or defend ourselves from the bison, mammoth or bear chasing us.

In modern days, where stress is chronic and cortisol levels are therefore consistently elevated, this excess glucose inhibits fat utilisation. Read that again.

Cortisol levels can be tested via a simple salivary test, and is most useful for those experiencing fat-loss barriers, particularly when their nutrition and lifestyle strategies are already dialled in.

Time to commit to meditation?

11 THE SNACKING MYTH

Another of the big food myths is that 'you need to eat every two hours to speed up your metabolism'. It may surprise you to hear that an efficient metabolism is actually a function of your satiety, created by LCHF. It's normal to feel overwhelmed initially, especially if you are a serial snacker, but with LCHF it is more than possible to only need three meals per day. After more than a decade of working in the weight-loss industry, I have found that this is one of the biggest change catalysts for most people. Eating every two hours is stressful, expensive and one of the big contributors to disordered eating. Not being bound by your appetite or the clock, however, is food freedom.

Here's why you need to use satiety as your biggest indicator:

1   When your meal provides five or more hours of energy, the composition is ideal. When you build your plate from predominantly non-starchy vegetables, quality protein and good fats, you are optimising nutrient density and opening up a fantastic fat-burning opportunity, meal to meal, as your blood sugar is stable and your insulin remains low.

2   Satiety allows for digestive ease and for energy to be used elsewhere, rather than constant digestion, which, as you now know, is a process that requires significantly large amounts of energy. Many people with poor digestion experience significant improvements by decreasing their meal frequency.

3   You learn how to eat intuitively rather than by the clock. No longer are you force-feeding yourself because you have been told you must eat frequently. It is actually possible to not need to snack when you are in control of your physiology, rather than letting it be in control of you.

So if you want porridge for breakfast (and feel it works for you), add nuts, seeds and berries to increase the nutrient density and blood sugar control. It's still not the perfect choice, as you're missing vegetables and a full serve of protein, but you could also be doing far worse. Rice cakes on occasions are fine, but add tuna, avocado and tomato rather than simply Vegemite or jam.

One thing I do want you to consider is that your meal frequency is relative to your eating window. What this means is that in a shorter eating window (i.e. when breakfast is later and/or dinner is earlier) you will need fewer meals than during a longer eating window (i.e. when breakfast is earlier and/or dinner is later).

Regardless, satiety is essential. If any of your current choices do not allow for five or more hours of satiety, please adjust your meals slightly by adding non-starchy vegetables and good fats first. Remember that the best choices always come off a tree, out of the ground or from an animal.

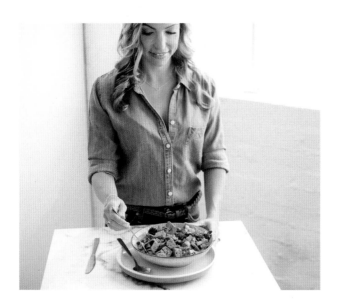

12 THE SATURATED-FAT HEART HEALTH MYTH

For five decades, health authorities have been telling us that saturated fat increases the risk of heart disease. But did you know that this theory has never been proved?

HOW DID THIS MYTH HAPPEN?

As we have discussed, a key proponent in the trajectory of our dietary guidelines was Ancel Keys, who cherry-picked data and noted a correlation between increased saturated fat consumption and heart disease. But we all know that correlation doesn't equal causation, right? You also can't exclude the data from fourteen countries simply because it doesn't fit your hypotheses. Thank goodness science has come a long way in the last five decades!

THE FACTS ABOUT SATURATED FATS AND HEART DISEASE

Saturated fats do not cause heart disease. We discussed the results of the 2010 meta-analysis that clearly state that there is 'no significant evidence for concluding that dietary saturated fat is associated with an increased risk of heart disease'.

It is also important to note that much of the initial research was conducted on rabbits, whose natural diet does not include cholesterol-containing food. Our cholesterol metabolism is essential for human life and, of course, vastly different to that of rabbits. Prior to the industrial revolution, saturated fat was the most prominent source of fat in the human diet. Our ancestors may have died young, but it certainly wasn't due to the consumption of margarine, seed oils, fried foods or refined sugar.

Dietary cholesterol only raises blood levels by 1 to 2 per cent, so its effect is only ever going to be mild. The even better news is that saturated fat actually exerts a positive influence on our high-density lipoprotein (HDL). The role of HDL is to transport cholesterol away from our arteries and towards the liver, where it may be either excreted or reused. Cholesterol is essential to human life – without cholesterol, we would die – and so our bodies have developed elaborate mechanisms to manufacture it, to make sure we always have enough.

THE BENEFITS OF SATURATED FATS

Saturated fats provide an abundance of health, and heart health, benefits. Lauric and stearic acids (found in saturated fats) help to regulate cholesterol levels and reduce lipoprotein A, a known risk factor for heart disease. Caprylic acid (found in MCT and coconut oil) has many antibacterial and antiviral properties, providing essential immune support. Saturated fats act as 'nervous system insulation', decreasing your susceptibility to internal and external stress. Not only is your brain predominantly made from saturated fat, but saturated fat provides the building blocks for our cell membranes and hormones, and also acts as a carrier for our fat-soluble vitamins A, D, E and K. Pretty essential, huh? Saturated fat is a concentrated source of energy and therefore has steadying effects on blood sugar and insulin. These are the keys to energy, satiety, mental clarity, cognition and weight control.

THE BEST SOURCES OF SATURATED FATS

Saturated fats are found in coconut oil, MCT oil, butter, ghee, beef fat, lamb fat, shellfish and in full-fat dairy foods – milk, cream and cheese. Choose from these. In case you haven't already, throw your low-fat products in the bin, please! If you choose to drink dairy, choose full-fat, unpasteurised and organic wherever possible.

To turn skim milk white, it is often fortified with powdered skim milk, which is liquid sprayed under heat and high pressure – a process that oxidises the cholesterol. In animal studies, oxidised cholesterol triggers a host of biological changes leading to plaque formation in the arteries and heart disease. Need I say more?

THE TRUTH ABOUT CHOLESTEROL

Cholesterol is the major component of our cell walls, the precursor to vitamin D, vital for proper neurological functioning and, importantly, the precursor to hormones including our sex hormones. The greatest amount of cholesterol does not come from dietary sources but from our liver, which produces cholesterol at the rate of approximately 1–2 grams per day.

As we have discussed, more than forty years ago the concept of cholesterol's impact upon cardiovascular disease emerged, and the misguided war on cholesterol began. We now, however, know the truth: inflammation, not cholesterol, causes heart disease.

Instead of examining total cholesterol from a lipid panel, the blood markers we should be using are:

- TC:HDL-C – where <3.5 is ideal
- Triglycerides – where <1.0 mmol/L is ideal
- C-reactive protein – where <1.0 mmol/L is ideal
- Homocysteine – where 7.0-7.5 mmol/L is ideal
  (also indicative of methylation status)

WHAT ABOUT STATINS?

In the 1950s, drug company scientists discovered the biochemical pathway to cholesterol synthesis, and the now trillion-dollar statin industry began. Statins are a class of drugs that lower cholesterol in the blood by reducing the production of cholesterol by the liver. When statins are administered in doses sufficient to compromise this synthesis of cholesterol, it is inevitable that the nutritional uptake required for cellular function is compromised. In the past few years, the true legacy of statin drugs has emerged. It is time to acknowledge their severe overprescription and re-evaluate their usage.

WHAT YOU NEED TO KNOW:

- Statins are a class of drugs that lower cholesterol in the blood by reducing the production of cholesterol by the liver.
- Yes, our liver produces cholesterol, at approximately 1–2 grams per day.
- Total cholesterol is not the cause of the disease, inflammation is.
- Dietary saturated fat is not associated with an increased risk of heart disease.
- Low-fat diets do nothing to control your disease risk, but they will make you hungry, fat, hormonally imbalanced and inflamed.

WHAT ARE THE SIDE EFFECTS OF STATINS?

The highest concentration (25 per cent) of cholesterol in the body is found in the brain. When cholesterol production is blocked, the side effects can be disastrous. The potential side effects of statin usage include confusion, paranoia, disorientation, depression, memory loss and dementia. Multiple studies have shown that statins decrease mitochondrial function (our energy powerhouses) and coenzyme Q10 (CoQ10) levels, which can lead to muscular weakness, instability, fatigue and muscle aches and pains.

Please note: There are some cases where statins can be beneficial; a cardiologist will advise you. What we do know is that there are effective strategies to assist patients who require statin therapy, including CoQ10 supplementation. This is specifically important for those people who want to participate in exercise but are limited due to the drug side effects.

TAKE-HOME MESSAGES:

- Cholesterol is not the problem. We do not need to artificially lower a vital substance that virtually every cell in our bodies naturally produces and requires to function optimally.
- From a blood lipid test, high total low-density lipoprotein (LDL) cholesterol is not the most important factor, but rather it's the size of the LDL particles that counts.
- Low TC-HDL-C indicates minimal small LDL particles and a reduced risk of heart disease.
- High-carbohydrate diets and the presence of insulin are responsible for small LDL particles.
- Statin drugs do nothing to change LDL particle size.
- Statins have the ability to impair adaptation to exercise due to pain, fatigue, decreased improvements in performance and increased recovery time.
- In the small percentage of cases where statins are necessary, they should be co-prescribed with a high-quality coenzyme Q10 supplementation.

13 THE LCHF KITCHEN

PANTRY BASICS

Stock your kitchen with these staples first, and getting started will be easy.

- nut milk
- almond flour
- coconut flour
- chia seeds
- coconut oil
- MCT oil
- raw cacao
- stevia

NUT MILK

Nut milk is a fantastic dairy-free alternative to pasteurised dairy. Great examples include almond and macadamia milk. If buying off the shelf, make sure you check the ingredients list and avoid sugar and products with more than five ingredients. You can also make these milks at home.

Why not cow's milk?

The reality is that the majority of dairy products are highly processed via a process referred to as pasteurisation. Pasteurised dairy products are subjected to high temperatures to destroy impurities. This simultaneously destroys the nutritious constituents. The truth is that the calcium actually becomes insoluble, the vitamin C is damaged, and many of the beneficial nutrients are destroyed.

Significantly, pasteurised dairy is potentially inflammatory. Inflammation makes the body acidic, which the body then attempts to neutralise. In order to do this, calcium is leeched from the bones, causing decreased calcium levels and potentially osteoporosis in the longer term. You have been told for decades to drink milk for strong bones, but for natural and nutrient-dense options, please prioritise dark leafy greens, sardines, sesame seeds, almonds, celery, rhubarb and oranges.

In the case of skim milk, it is often fortified with powdered skim milk, which is liquid sprayed under heat and high pressure, a process that oxidises the cholesterol. Low-fat yoghurt is mostly high in sugar and, again, depleted of nutrients due to the pasteurisation process. Throw your low-fat products in the bin, please.

ALMOND FLOUR

Almond flour is one of the best substitutes for wheat available. It is easy to make and cook with, and delicious. Nutritionally, almond flour is full of heart-healthy monounsaturated fats, and high in vitamin E, magnesium and fibre. Low in carbohydrates and sugars, it's perfect to avoid the 'wheat belly' or 'muffin top' associated with some common gluten-free substitutes, like potato starch and corn starch.

Flour v. meal

Both are available at your local health-food store and in the baking aisle of the supermarket. The difference is usually that almond meal is ground whole almonds, whereas almond flour is blanched almonds with the skin removed. Both are interchangeable in most recipes, but the texture will be different, so please keep this in mind.

To make your own, simply blend raw almonds in the food processor. Yes, it really is that easy.

COCONUT FLOUR

Coconut flour is a must-have addition to your pantry. It is not only gluten free, grain free and low carbohydrate, but also extremely nutritious. Here's why:

- Coconut flour is 14 per cent coconut oil, a medium-chain triglyceride (MCT) that is easily digested and readily absorbed by the liver. MCTs are used as a direct source of energy by our brains and muscles rather than for fat storage (which is what happens when you consume trans fats, amongst other things). Studies show that the consumption of coconut oil can assist in calorie burning, fat oxidation and reduced food intake, and as a result, weight loss.
- Coconut flour is made up of 58 per cent dietary fibre, and is therefore fantastic for blood sugar control, satiety and curbing cravings, all of which are essential for weight management. It is one of the biggest nutrition myths that wholegrains and cereals are required for fibre, when fruit and vegetables are the highest sources of fibre known to man.
- Coconut flour is rich in protein – great for satiety, blood sugar control, immunity and recovery from exercise, just to start.
- Coconut flour contains manganese, a vitamin that is essential for the thyroid gland, which is the regulator of our metabolism, growth and energy expenditure.

Coconut flour: tips and tricks

- Due to its density, unfortunately you cannot simply substitute coconut flour for other flours. A useful guide is to start with ⅓ cup for every cup of 'normal' flour.
- Coconut flour and almond flour work really well together. If the density of coconut flour on its own is not to your liking, you can modify it by replacing half the quantity with almond flour. Adding a small amount to your favourite recipe is a great place to start, and should not change the liquid requirements or texture too much.

- Coconut flour is not just for sweet treats. It makes a great low-carb coating for schnitzels, or can be used as a breadcrumb replacement for coating meatballs. It does have a sweeter flavour than conventional flours, though, so keep that in mind when cooking for others.
- Coconut flour is one of the more expensive flours, so you can consider shopping online and/or buying in bulk to save money.

CHIA SEEDS

Chia seeds are truly one of nature's superfoods. Their high omega-3 and natural fibre content makes them fantastic for blood sugar control, which is the key to satiety, energy and weight management. They are a complete protein, providing all of our essential amino acids – which is actually quite rare from a vegetarian source. Chia seeds are high in calcium, making them a great dairy-free alternative for bone health.

How to use them
- Add to smoothies (just soak in liquid for 5 minutes first).
- Use in raw treats for extra satiety and crunch.
- Add to homemade cereal or granola.
- Make a chia pudding: 3 tablespoons soaked overnight in your choice of milk, then topped with nuts, seeds and coconut yoghurt prior to serving.
- Try this 'chia egg' as a fantastic vegan egg replacement.

'CHIA EGG'

1 tablespoon chia seeds
3 tablespoons water

In a small bowl, soak chia seeds in water for 5 minutes. Use as you would egg in baked goods. If a recipe calls for 4 eggs, use 4 'chia eggs'. So simple.

COCONUT AND MCT OIL

Coconut oil has a high saturated fat content and, more specifically, is high in MCTs – 66 per cent, in fact. MCTs are extracted and isolated from pure coconut oil and have increased in popularity in recent years. They are mostly available online or from your local health-food store.

In contrast to long-chain triglycerides, MCTs are easily digested and readily absorbed by the liver, and are therefore a direct source of energy. This means fuel for our brain and muscles, rather than fat storage. Studies have shown that the consumption of MCTs can assist in calorie burning, fat oxidation and reduced food intake, and as a result, weight loss.

Additional health benefits include:

- Improved insulin sensitivity (and therefore type 2 diabetes control)
- Enhanced digestion and the alleviation of digestive disorders such as irritable bowel syndrome
- Immunity – coconut oil consists of lauric, caprylic and capric acids, all of which have fantastic antibacterial and antiviral properties

RAW CACAO

Raw cacao is nature's super bean. Due to its extremely high ORAC score (a measure of antioxidant quantity), it is actually classed as a 'super-antioxidant'. It helps to prevent cellular damage, protect the heart and naturally fight the ageing process.

Cacao is also a great source of flavonoids, essential fatty acids and magnesium – all of which help with metabolism, premenstrual symptoms, heart function, blood pressure and lowering chronic disease risk. Raw cacao contains naturally occurring theobromine, which acts as a mild, non-addictive stimulant that some believe can treat depression. Studies show that theobromine assists the brain to produce more anandamide, a 'feel-good' neurotransmitter.

Please note: Cacao is not the same as cocoa (which is highly processed and low in nutrition) and is always best in its raw form, without the added sugar that most commercial chocolates contain. Opt for 85 per cent dark chocolate when you can, and try our Healthy MCT Hot Chocolate (see recipe page 242) to assist with sugar cravings and to aid satiety after a meal.

STEVIA

Stevia is our preferred LCHF sweetener. It is a naturally occurring herb with zero calories and negligible blood sugar impact. It is important to understand that anything sweet can stimulate the desire for more sweet foods and that even though it is the best option, there is some research to show that it can interfere, via the hypothalamus, with insulin levels and therefore hunger, cravings and body weight management. Use it sparingly in your treats by all means, but it should not be considered an 'everyday food'.

LCHF MEAL PLANS

We've dived into the science, we've explored the food pyramid and our food guidelines, we've broken down the archaic dogma, exposed many food myths and started exploring new ingredients. So where to next?

It's time for you to experience the benefits first-hand! I've provided four 14-day meal plans to cater for different goals: fat loss, diabetes management, endurance fuelling, and fasting. All of these meal plans are simple to follow and, as far as is possible, use leftovers for lunch the next day. 'Cook once, eat twice' will soon become your new mantra, and you will learn how much it contributes positively to making your newfound lifestyle sustainable, cost-effective and stress-free. You also have more than 150 LCHF recipes to try, all of which contain minimal ingredients and are free from refined sugars, refined seed oils, trans fats, poor-quality dairy and gluten. Remember, this is how to supercharge your metabolism and optimise your health, energy levels, hormones, performance, recovery and longevity. Enjoy!

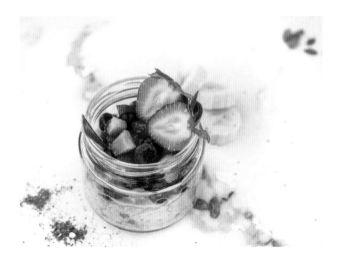

14-DAY FAT LOSS MEAL PLAN

WEEK 1	BREAKFAST	LUNCH	DINNER
M	Carrot Cake Chia Pudding	Green Chicken Curry with Cauliflower Rice	Lamb Cutlets + Super-easy Side Salad
T	Gluten-free & Sugar-free Granola	Lamb Cutlets + Super-easy Side Salad*	Pumpkin & Feta Chicken Salad
W	Breakfast Antioxidant Smoothie#1	Pumpkin & Feta Chicken Salad*	Chicken Satay Stir-fry with Cauliflower Rice
T	Mushroom, Spinach & Asparagus Omelette	Chicken Satay Stir-fry with Cauliflower Rice*	Oven-baked Fish + Spinach & Fennel Salad
F	Meal in a Jar	Oven-baked Fish + Spinach & Fennel Salad*	Mushroom Burgers with Kale Chips
S	Eggs, Haloumi, Spinach & Tomato	Chicken Satay Stir-fry with Cauliflower Rice*	Shepherd's Pie with Pumpkin Mash & Buttered Greens
S	Easy Green Omelette + Almost Paleo Vegie Bread	Shepherd's Pie with Pumpkin Mash + Buttered Greens*	Salmon Fillet with Roasted Brussels Sprouts & Fennel Salad

^ Prepare the night before   * Leftovers

WEEK 2	BREAKFAST	LUNCH	DINNER
M	Gluten-free & Sugar-free Granola	Salmon Fillet with Roasted Brussels Sprouts & Fennel Salad*	Chicken Abundance Bowl
T	Pumpkin, Feta & Bacon Frittata^	Chicken Abundance Bowl*	Zucchini 'Spaghetti' Bolognese
W	Meal in a Jar	Zucchini 'Spaghetti' Bolognese*	Oven-baked Fish + Steamed Broccolini with Feta
T	Pumpkin, Feta & Bacon Frittata*	Oven-baked Fish + Steamed Broccolini with Feta* + Cauliflower Mash^	Low Carb Seafood 'Fried Rice'
F	Mushroom, Spinach & Asparagus Omelette + Almost Paleo Vegie Bread	Low Carb Seafood 'Fried Rice'*	Clean Chicken Parma with Zucchini Chips
S	LCHF Breakfast Burrito	Chicken Broccolini Beauty	Clean Snags with Warm Broccoli Salad
S	Meal in a Jar	Pumpkin & Feta Chicken Salad	Grass-fed Steak + Super-easy Side Salad

^ Prepare the night before   * Leftovers

LOW CARB HEALTHY FAT NUTRITION

14-DAY DIABETES MANAGEMENT PLAN

BREAKFAST	LUNCH	DINNER	WEEK 1
LCHF Frittata with Avocado^	Zucchini 'Spaghetti' Bolognese^	Salmon with Buttered Greens & Cauliflower Mash	M
Green Machine Smoothie	Salmon with Buttered Greens & Cauliflower Mash*	Clean Snags with Pumpkin Mash & Asparagus	T
Berry & Coconut Chia Pudding	Clean Snags with Pumpkin Mash & Asparagus*	Chicken Thighs + Simple Tomato Salad	W
LCHF Frittata with Avocado^	Chicken Thighs + Simple Tomato Salad*	Low Carb Seafood 'Fried Rice'	T
Mixed Berry & Tahini Smoothie	Low Carb Seafood 'Fried Rice'*	Steak with Zucchini & Brussels Sprouts Salad	F
Low Carb Breakfast Hash	Pumpkin & Feta Chicken Salad	Mexican Beef Tortillas	S
Eggs, Haloumi, Spinach & Tomato	Mexican Beef Tortillas	Chicken Satay Stir-fry with Cauliflower Rice	S

^ Prepare the night before   * Leftovers

BREAKFAST	LUNCH	DINNER	WEEK 2
Simple Eggs & Broccoli	Chicken Satay Stir-fry with Cauliflower Rice*	Shepherd's Pie with Pumpkin Mash + Steamed Broccolini with Feta	M
Green Machine Smoothie	Shepherd's Pie with Pumpkin Mash + Steamed Broccolini with Feta*	Grass-fed Steak + Super-easy Side Salad	T
Carrot Cake Chia Pudding	Grass-fed Steak + Super-easy Side Salad*	Salmon Fillet with Roasted Brussels Sprouts & Fennel Salad*	W
Breakfast Antioxidant Smoothie#2	Salmon Fillet with Roasted Brussels Sprouts & Fennel Salad*	Chicken Thighs + Simple Greek Salad	T
LSA & Chia Pudding with Raspberries	Chicken Thighs + Simple Greek Salad*	Oven-baked Fish + Beetroot, Goat's Feta & Walnut Salad	F
Egg-free Breakfast Hash	Mushroom, Spinach & Asparagus Omelette	Paleo Burgers	S
LCHF Breakfast Burrito	Chicken Broccolini Beauty	Zucchini 'Spaghetti' Bolognese	S

^ Prepare the night before   * Leftovers

14-DAY ENDURANCE MEAL PLAN

WEEK 1	BREAKFAST	LUNCH	DINNER
M	Gluten-free & Sugar-free Granola	Lamb & Cauliflower Salad^	Chicken Abundance Bowl
T	Breakfast Antioxidant Smoothie#1	Chicken Abundance Bowl*	Zucchini 'Spaghetti' Bolognese
W	Gluten-free & Sugar-free Granola	Zucchini 'Spaghetti' Bolognese*	Oven-baked Fish + Broccoli & Kale Salad
T	Three-egg Omelette	Oven-baked Fish + Broccoli & Kale Salad*	Steak with Rocket, Walnut & Pear Salad
F	Berry & Coconut Chia Pudding	Steak with Rocket, Walnut & Pear Salad*	Vegie Abundance Bowl
S	Lower Carb Smoothie Bowl	Rainbow Omelette	Paleo Burgers#1
S	Breakfast Salad with Boiled Egg	Chicken Caesar Salad	Lamb Stir-fry with Broccoli Rice

^ Prepare the night before * Leftovers
After a high-intensity training session, add 1 serve of complex carbohydrates.

WEEK 2	BREAKFAST	LUNCH	DINNER
M	Chorizo & Goat's Feta Omelette + Almost Paleo Vegie Bread^	Lamb Stir-fry with Broccoli Rice*	Chicken Caesar Salad*
T	Blueberry & Macadamia Smoothie	Chicken Caesar Salad*	Green LCHF 'Pasta'
W	Gluten-free & Sugar-free Granola	Green LCHF 'Pasta'*	Salmon on Pea Mash
T	Three-egg Omelette + Almost Paleo Vegie Bread^	Salmon on Pea Mash*	Green Chicken Curry with Cauliflower Rice
F	Blueberry & Macadamia Smoothie	Green Chicken Curry with Cauliflower Rice*	Lamb Cutlets + Simple Greek Salad
S	LCHF Breakfast Burrito	Chicken Broccolini Beauty	Baked Fish with Tahini
S	Green Baked Eggs	Blueberry & Macadamia Smoothie	Gluten-free Chicken Schnitz with Buttered Greens

^ Prepare the night before * Leftovers
After high-intensity training, add 1 serve of complex carbohydrates.

14-DAY FASTING MEAL PLAN

BREAKFAST	LUNCH	SNACKS	DINNER	WEEK 1
Breakfast Antioxidant Smoothie	Clean Snags with Warm Broccoli Salad^		Baked Fish with Tahini	M
Melrose MCT Coffee	Baked Fish with Tahini*	2 × celery sticks with nut butter	Chicken Abundance Bowl #2	T
Gluten-free & Sugar-free Granola	Chicken Abundance Bowl #2*		Paleo Burgers #2	W
Anti-Inflammatory MCT Coffee	Paleo Burgers #2*	1 × 'On-the-go' Muffin^	Salmon Fillet with Roasted Brussels Sprouts & Fennel Salad	T
Gluten-free & Sugar-free Granola	Salmon Fillet with Roasted Brussels Sprouts & Fennel Salad*		Clean Chicken Parma with Buttered Greens	F
Green Baked Eggs	Clean Chicken Parma with Buttered Greens*		Steak with Rocket, Walnut & Pear Salad	S
Easy Green Omelette	Steak with Rocket, Walnut & Pear Salad*		Low Carb Seafood 'Fried Rice'	S

^ Prepare the night before   * Leftovers

BREAKFAST	LUNCH	SNACKS	DINNER	WEEK 2
Hormonal-balancing MCT Coffee	Low Carb Seafood 'Fried Rice'*	1 × 'On-the-go' Muffin^	Salmon with Buttered Greens & Cauliflower Mash	M
Carrot Cake Chia Pudding	Salmon with Buttered Greens & Cauliflower Mash*		Clean Snags with Pumpkin Mash & Asparagus	T
Melrose MCT Coffee	Clean Snags with Pumpkin Mash & Asparagus*	2 × celery sticks with nut butter	Vegie Abundance Bowl	W
Carrot Cake Chia Pudding	Vegie Abundance Bowl*		Chicken Stir-fry with Cauliflower Rice	T
Scrambled Green Eggs	Chicken Stir-fry with Cauliflower Rice*		Steak with Zucchini & Brussels Sprouts Salad	F
Baked Zucchini Pancakes	Steak with Zucchini & Brussels Sprouts Salad*		Mexican Beef Tortillas	S
Low Carb Breakfast Hash	Mexican Beef Tortillas*		Mushroom Burgers with Kale Chips	S

^ Prepare the night before   * Leftovers

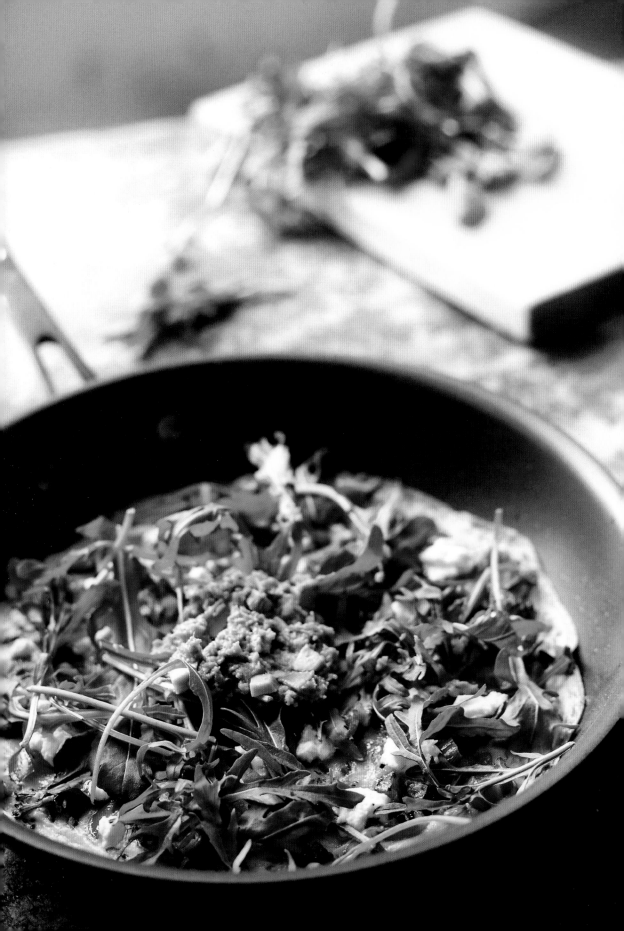

BREAKFAST

The meal you choose in the morning shapes your entire day. With your LCHF breakfasts you'll be well satiated and ready for the day ahead.

RAINBOW OMELETTE

SERVES (F)(M) 1   PREP : 10 MINUTES   COOK : 15 MINUTES

'Eating the rainbow' is a huge part of your LCHF template, and this omelette really ticks all the boxes. To fast-track the preparation time, pick a dinner recipe with roasted pumpkin the night before and put some aside for the next morning. To me, pumpkin roasted in coconut oil and sea salt is so delicious that it almost feels indulgent!

½ cup finely diced pumpkin
sea salt and pepper, to taste
1 tablespoon cold-pressed
    extra-virgin coconut oil
2 free-range eggs
1 rasher pasture-raised bacon,
    diced / 2 rashers pasture-
    raised bacon, diced
½ red capsicum, finely diced
1 bunch broccolini, roughly
    chopped
4 cherry tomatoes, diced /
    6 cherry tomatoes, diced
1 cup spinach leaves
1 tablespoon roughly
    chopped chives
30g goat's feta
20g rocket leaves
½ avocado, mashed

1 Preheat oven to 180°C and line a baking tray with baking paper.

2 Place pumpkin on the tray, season with salt, drizzle with half the oil and roast for 10 minutes, or until golden.

3 Whisk eggs in a bowl until well combined. Set aside.

4 Heat a small ovenproof frying pan over medium heat and add remaining oil. Sauté bacon and capsicum until softened. Add broccolini and tomatoes and continue to sauté. Add spinach and stir until wilted.

5 Toss through pumpkin and chives, ensuring all ingredients are well combined, and season well with salt and pepper.

6 Pour the egg over the bacon and vegetables, and sprinkle with feta. When the eggs are starting to set, transfer to the oven until cooked to your liking.

7 Season to taste again before serving, and top with rocket leaves and avocado.

(F) MACROS Cals : 612   CHO : 18g   P : 28g   Fat : 50g
(M) MACROS Cals : 785   CHO : 33g   P : 43g   Fat : 56g

SIMPLE EGGS & BROCCOLI

SERVES Ⓕ Ⓜ 1   PREP : 5 MINUTES   COOK : 10 MINUTES

I still remember the first time I made this recipe. So simple, yet such a great way to get vegetables in at breakfast. Broccoli is one of my favourite non-starchy vegetables – not only is it versatile, it's terrific for your liver, digestive system, immune system and bone strength.

2 cups broccoli florets
2 free-range eggs /
  3 free-range eggs
1 tablespoon cold-pressed
  extra-virgin coconut oil /
  **2 tablespoons cold-pressed
  extra-virgin coconut oil**
½ avocado, diced /
  1 avocado, diced
30g goat's feta
sea salt and pepper, to taste

1 Bring a small saucepan of water to the boil. Place broccoli in a colander or steamer basket, cover with a lid and steam for 4–5 minutes. Transfer to a serving plate.

2 Fry eggs in the coconut oil and place on top of the broccoli.

3 Top with avocado, sprinkle with feta, and season well with salt and pepper.

Ⓕ MACROS Cals : **532** CHO : **21g**· P : **26g** Fat : **48g**
Ⓜ MACROS Cals : **860** CHO : **27g** P : **33g** Fat : **71g**

LCHF FRITTATA WITH AVOCADO

SERVES Ⓕ Ⓜ 4   PREP : 10 MINUTES   COOK : 30 MINUTES

Frittatas are a great breakfast option, especially mid-week when you are time-poor. I prefer to make mine on a Sunday and store portions in glass containers for the week ahead. The addition of chorizo here is a real treat – just make sure you choose a quality brand that is pasture-raised and without added nasties.

**1 teaspoon cold-pressed
  extra-virgin coconut oil**
10 free-range eggs /
  12 free-range eggs
¼ teaspoon sea salt
1 teaspoon chilli flakes
200ml coconut cream
1 large zucchini, grated
1 large carrot, grated
**250g pasture-raised
  chorizo, cubed**

TO SERVE, PER PERSON
1 medium avocado, sliced

1 Preheat oven to 180°C and lightly grease a ceramic or glass baking dish with coconut oil.

2 In a large bowl, whisk eggs with salt and chilli. Add coconut cream and whisk further until well combined.

3 Add grated vegetables and chorizo and combine.

4 Pour frittata mix into the baking dish and bake for 30 minutes, or until cooked throughout.

5 Cut into 4 portions, serve with avocado, and enjoy.

Ⓕ MACROS Cals : **513** CHO : **9g** P : **30g** Fat : **40g**
Ⓜ MACROS Cals : **712** CHO : **23g** P : **35g** Fat : **52g**

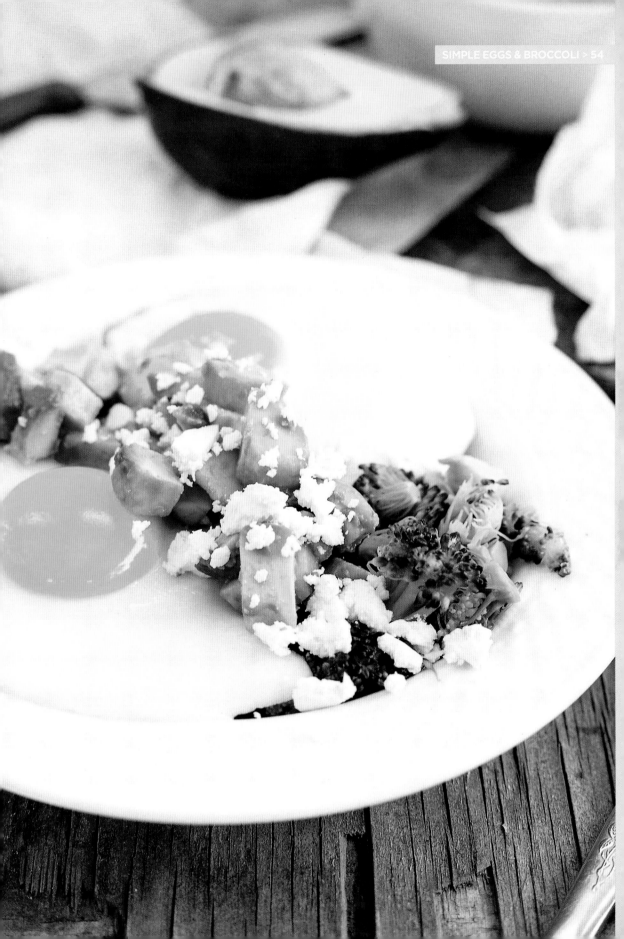

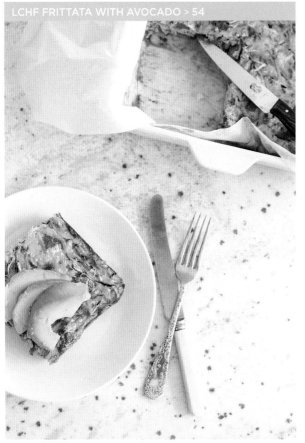

LCHF FRITTATA WITH AVOCADO > 54

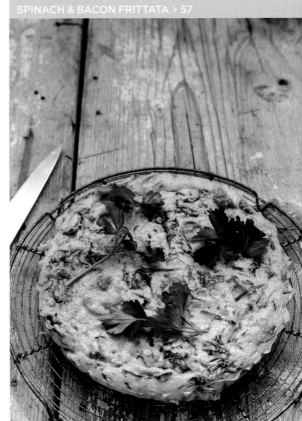

SPINACH & BACON FRITTATA > 57

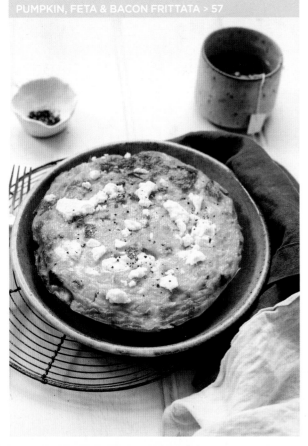

PUMPKIN, FETA & BACON FRITTATA > 57

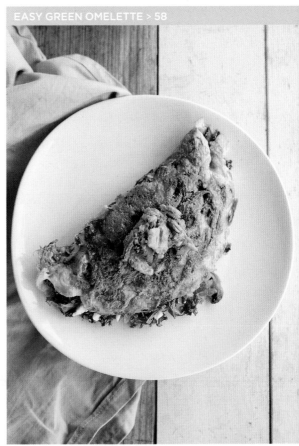

EASY GREEN OMELETTE > 58

SPINACH & BACON FRITTATA

SERVES Ⓕ Ⓜ 4   PREP : 10 MINUTES   COOK : 35 MINUTES

1 tablespoon cold-pressed
  extra-virgin coconut oil
200g spinach leaves
3 rashers pasture-raised
  bacon, diced / 4 rashers
  pasture-raised bacon, diced
1 zucchini, grated
1 carrot, grated
¼ bunch parsley, roughly
  chopped
6 free-range eggs /
  10 free-range eggs
⅓ cup coconut flour
1 tablespoon macadamia oil
200ml coconut cream
125g cherry tomatoes, sliced
sea salt and pepper, to taste

1 Preheat oven to 180°C and line a 30cm × 20cm baking
   tray with baking paper.

2 Heat coconut oil in a frypan over medium heat and sauté
   spinach for 2–3 minutes, or until wilted. Set aside.

3 Sauté bacon until golden. Set aside.

4 Place grated zucchini and carrot in a large bowl and stir
   in parsley, spinach and bacon.

5 In a separate bowl, whisk eggs well, until bubbles appear.

6 Stir coconut flour into eggs, then mix in quickly with
   the vegetable mixture to ensure all ingredients are well
   combined. Add macadamia oil and coconut cream and
   stir well.

7 Pour mixture into the prepared baking tin, top with the
   cherry tomato slices and season well with salt and pepper.

8 Bake for 25–30 minutes, or until golden and firm to press.

Ⓕ MACROS Cals : **353** CHO : **13g** P : **15g** Fat : **28g**
Ⓜ MACROS Cals : **583** CHO : **18g** P : **32g** Fat : **42g**

PUMPKIN, FETA & BACON FRITTATA

SERVES Ⓕ Ⓜ 4   PREP : 10 MINUTES   COOK : 40 MINUTES

1 teaspoon cold-pressed
  extra-virgin coconut oil /
  1 tablespoon cold-pressed
  extra-virgin coconut oil
400g pumpkin, diced
4 rashers pasture-raised
  bacon, diced
12 free-range eggs
¼ teaspoon sea salt
1 teaspoon chilli flakes
200ml coconut cream /
  400ml coconut cream
100g goat's feta, crumbled

1 Preheat oven to 180°C and lightly grease a ceramic or glass
   baking dish with half the coconut oil.

2 Heat a frypan over medium heat and add remaining oil. Add
   pumpkin and stir-fry until golden. Add bacon and continue to
   cook for a further 3–4 minutes, or until golden. Set aside.

3 In a large bowl, whisk eggs with salt and chilli. Add coconut
   cream and whisk further until well combined.

4 Add pumpkin and bacon mixture, along with the feta, and
   stir well to combine.

5 Transfer to the baking dish and bake for 30 minutes, or until
   cooked through.

6 Allow to cool before cutting and serving.

Ⓕ MACROS Cals : **511** CHO : **11g** P : **45g** Fat : **36g**
Ⓜ MACROS Cals : **732** CHO : **13g** P : **45g** Fat : **59g**

EASY GREEN OMELETTE

SERVES (F) (M) 1   PREP : 5 MINUTES   COOK : 10 MINUTES

Omelettes are a staple of mine, and they are so versatile, too. While this Easy Green Omelette is usually enjoyed as a breakfast recipe, I often eat it for lunch or dinner after a late night with clients.

2 free-range eggs /
  3 free-range eggs
½ bunch broccolini, roughly
  chopped
2 button mushrooms, chopped
2 rashers pasture-raised bacon,
  diced
1 teaspoon cold-pressed
  extra-virgin coconut oil /
  2 teaspoons cold-pressed
  extra-virgin coconut oil
30g goat's feta
½ cup finely chopped kale
½ avocado, mashed /
  1 avocado, mashed
sea salt and pepper, to taste

1 In a large bowl, whisk eggs. Stir in broccolini, mushrooms and bacon.

2 Lightly grease a frypan with coconut oil and place over medium heat. Pour egg mix into the pan and cook until eggs start to set, or to your liking.

3 Sprinkle feta and kale over one half of the omelette. Gently fold the other half over the filling and cook for a further 1–2 minutes.

4 Serve omelette with avocado mash, and season with salt and pepper to taste.

(F) MACROS Cals : 676 CHO : 14g P : 32g Fat : 44g
(M) MACROS Cals : 742 CHO : 18g P : 38g Fat : 59g

EGGS, HALOUMI, SPINACH & TOMATO

SERVES (F) (M) 1   PREP : 5 MINUTES   COOK : 10 MINUTES

1 tablespoon cold-pressed
  extra-virgin coconut oil /
  2 tablespoons cold-pressed
  extra-virgin coconut oil
60g haloumi, cut into 5cm
  strips / 100g haloumi,
  cut into 5cm strips
2 free-range eggs /
  3 free-range eggs
1 tomato, halved
2 cups spinach leaves
1 slice of Almost Paleo Vegie
  Bread (see recipe page 206),
  for serving, optional
sea salt and pepper, to taste

1 Heat coconut oil in a small frypan over medium heat and cook haloumi for 2–3 minutes on each side, or until golden.

2 Remove haloumi from pan but retain fat, and fry eggs, tomato and spinach. Serve alongside haloumi and, if you like, toasted bread. Season with salt and pepper to taste.

(F) MACROS Cals : 502 CHO : 10g P : 27g Fat : 40g
(Ⓣ) MACROS Cals : 718 CHO : 21g P : 36g Fat : 56g
(M) MACROS Cals : 845 CHO : 12g P : 41g Fat : 69g
(Ⓣ) MACROS Cals : 1061 CHO : 23g P : 50g Fat : 85g

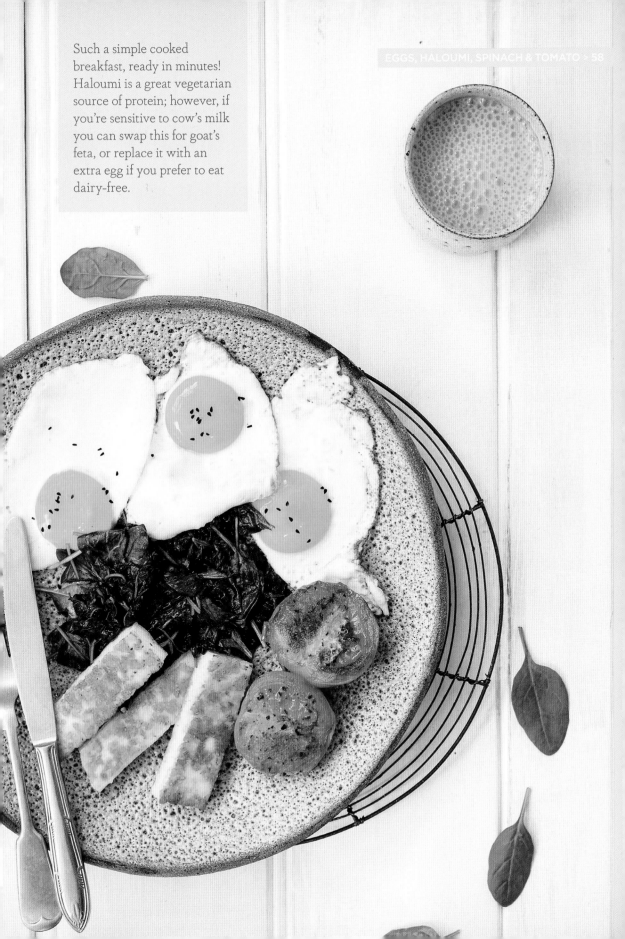

Such a simple cooked breakfast, ready in minutes! Haloumi is a great vegetarian source of protein; however, if you're sensitive to cow's milk you can swap this for goat's feta, or replace it with an extra egg if you prefer to eat dairy-free.

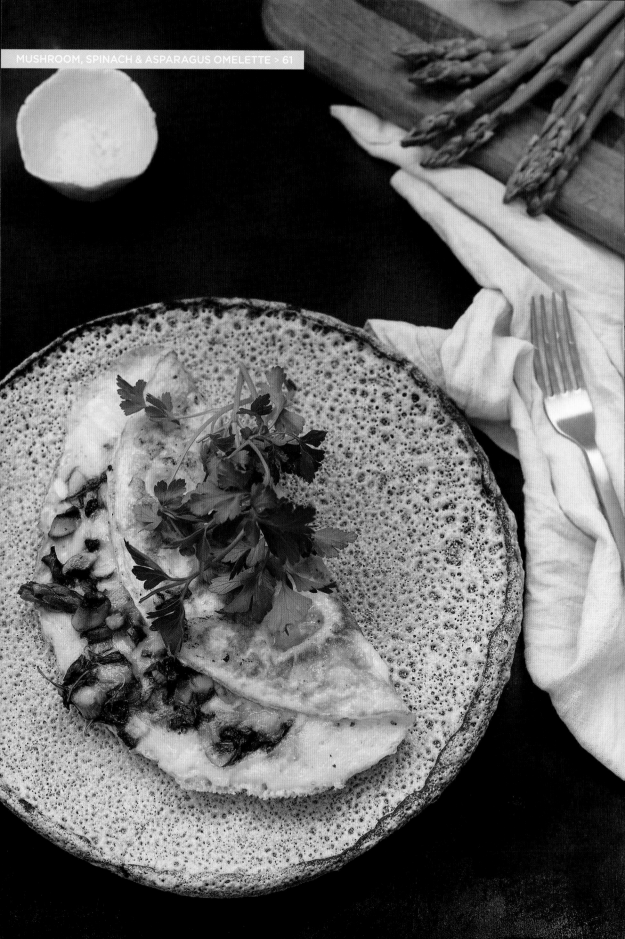

MUSHROOM, SPINACH & ASPARAGUS OMELETTE

SERVES Ⓕ Ⓜ 1   PREP : 5 MINUTES   COOK : 10 MINUTES

2 teaspoons cold-pressed
  extra-virgin coconut oil
2 button mushrooms, sliced
50g baby spinach leaves
2 asparagus spears, diced
3 free-range eggs
20g organic hard cheese,
  grated / 50g organic hard
  cheese, grated
2 tablespoons chopped fresh
  parsley
sea salt and pepper, to taste
1 slice of Almost Paleo Vegie
  Bread (see recipe page 206),
  for serving, optional

1   Place a non-stick frypan over medium heat, add oil and
    sauté mushrooms, spinach and asparagus. Set aside.

2   In a bowl, whisk together eggs with 2 tablespoons of
    water, pour into the pan and cook for a few minutes until
    egg starts to set.

3   Sprinkle mushrooms, spinach and asparagus over one half
    of the omelette. Top with cheese and parsley. Gently fold
    the other half of the omelette over the filling. Season with
    salt and pepper and serve with toasted bread, if you like.

Ⓕ	MACROS	Cals : 403	CHO : 5g	P : 26g	Fat : 31g
ⓘ	MACROS	Cals : 619	CHO : 16g	P : 35g	Fat : 47g
Ⓜ	MACROS	Cals : 556	CHO : 9g	P : 37g	Fat : 41g
ⓘ	MACROS	Cals : 772	CHO : 20g	P : 46g	Fat : 57g

THREE-EGG OMELETTE

SERVES Ⓕ Ⓜ 1   PREP : 5 MINUTES   COOK : 10 MINUTES

3 free-range eggs
1 teaspoon unsweetened
  coconut or almond milk /
  100ml unsweetened
  coconut or almond milk
1 tomato, diced
1 mushroom, diced
20g spinach leaves, finely
  chopped
½ teaspoon cold-pressed
  extra-virgin coconut oil /
  2 teaspoons cold-pressed
  extra-virgin coconut oil
20g goat's feta / 30g goat's feta
½ avocado, sliced / 1 avocado,
  sliced
1 slice of Almost Paleo Vegie
  Bread (see recipe page 206),
  for serving, optional
sea salt and pepper, to taste

1   In a large bowl, whisk eggs then stir in milk, tomato,
    mushroom and spinach.

2   Lightly grease a frypan with coconut oil and place over
    medium heat. Pour egg mix into the pan and cook
    until eggs start to set, or to your liking.

3   Sprinkle feta over one half of the omelette. Gently fold
    the other half over the feta.

4   Serve with avocado and, if you like, toasted bread. Season
    with salt and pepper.

Ⓕ	MACROS	Cals : 550	CHO : 11g	P : 27g	Fat : 44g
ⓘ	MACROS	Cals : 766	CHO : 22g	P : 36g	Fat : 60g
Ⓜ	MACROS	Cals : 890	CHO : 22g	P : 33g	Fat : 76g
ⓘ	MACROS	Cals : 1061	CHO : 33g	P : 42g	Fat : 92g

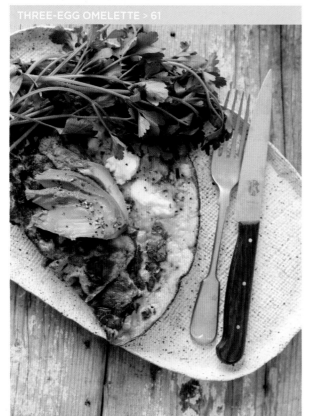
THREE-EGG OMELETTE > 61

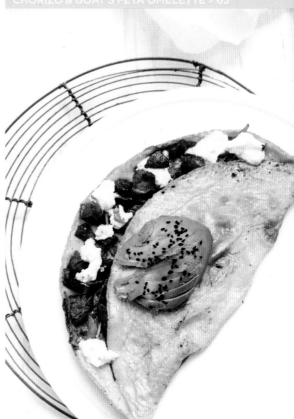
CHORIZO & GOAT'S FETA OMELETTE > 63

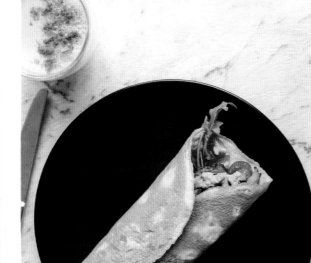
LCHF BREAKFAST BURRITO > 63

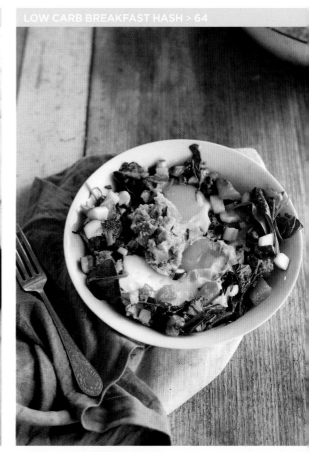
LOW CARB BREAKFAST HASH > 64

CHORIZO & GOAT'S FETA OMELETTE

SERVES Ⓕ Ⓜ 1   PREP : 5 MINUTES   COOK : 10 MINUTES

15g grass-fed butter /
   30g grass-fed butter
50g pasture-raised chorizo,
   finely diced / 100g pasture-
   raised chorizo, finely diced
2 free-range eggs / 3 free-range
   eggs
1 cup baby spinach leaves /
   2 cups baby spinach leaves
30g goat's feta
sea salt and pepper, to taste
½ avocado, sliced
1 slice of Almost Paleo Vegie
   Bread (see recipe page 206),
   for serving, optional

1 Heat a frypan over medium heat. Add half the butter and
   sauté chorizo for 3–4 minutes, or until golden. Set aside.

2 In a bowl, whisk eggs together with 1 tablespoon of water.

3 Add the remaining butter to the frypan and, once melted,
   pour in egg mixture and cook for a few minutes, until egg
   starts to set.

4 Sprinkle chorizo, spinach and feta over half the omelette.
   Cook on low heat for a further 2 minutes then gently fold
   the other half of the omelette over the filling. Cook for a
   further minute, or to your liking. Season well with salt and
   pepper, and serve with sliced avocado and toasted bread.

Ⓕ MACROS Cals : 575   CHO : 8g   P : 26g   Fat : 46g
☖ MACROS Cals : 791   CHO : 19g   P : 35g   Fat : 62g
Ⓜ MACROS Cals : 962   CHO : 10g   P : 42g   Fat : 83g
☖ MACROS Cals : 1178 CHO : 21g   P : 51g   Fat : 99g

LCHF BREAKFAST BURRITO

SERVES Ⓕ Ⓜ 1   PREP : 5 MINUTES   COOK : 10 MINUTES

You are going to love my spin on a breakfast burrito. Not only is it lower carbohydrate
but it is grain free, dairy free and nut free. I have no doubt that this will soon become
a new staple in your household.

1 rasher pasture-raised bacon /
   2 rashers pasture-raised
   bacon
2 free-range eggs / 3 free-range
   eggs
1 tablespoon cold-pressed
   extra-virgin coconut oil
¼ punnet cherry tomatoes
½ avocado / 1 avocado
50g rocket leaves
sea salt and pepper, to taste

1 Place a large frypan over medium heat and fry bacon until
   golden. Set aside.

2 In a bowl, whisk eggs until bubbles form.

3 Heat coconut oil in the frypan over low heat and ensure
   even coverage over the pan.

4 Pour in egg, making sure it covers the pan in a thin, even
   layer. Cook egg slowly, without flipping, for 6–8 minutes.

5 While the egg is cooking, dice tomatoes and mash avocado.

6 Slide the egg burrito onto a warmed plate and top with
   rocket, bacon, tomatoes and avocado. Season with salt and
   pepper, and fold gently as you would a burrito.

Ⓕ MACROS Cals : 469   CHO : 14g   P : 19g   Fat : 38g
Ⓜ MACROS Cals : 748   CHO : 20g   P : 37g   Fat : 60g

LOW CARB BREAKFAST HASH

SERVES (F) (M) 1   PREP : 5 MINUTES   COOK : 10 MINUTES

½ cup finely diced pumpkin
30g grass-fed butter
1 zucchini, finely diced
½ cup finely chopped broccoli
1 cup spinach leaves
2 free-range eggs
½ avocado, sliced /
  1 avocado, sliced
sea salt and pepper, to taste

1 Bring a small saucepan of water to the boil. Place pumpkin in a colander or steamer basket, cover with a lid and steam for 4–5 minutes.

2 Melt butter in a large frypan over medium heat, add pumpkin and cook until caramelised, stirring throughout.

3 Add zucchini and broccoli and sauté for 1–2 minutes, or until slightly softened. Add spinach and stir through well.

4 Make two holes in the mixture, crack an egg into each hole and cook until eggs are to your liking.

5 Remove from heat and transfer to a serving bowl. Top with avocado, season with salt and pepper, and enjoy.

(F) MACROS Cals : **628** CHO : **21g** P : **10g** Fat : **54g**
(M) MACROS Cals : **771** CHO : **33g** P : **22g** Fat : **64g**

EGG-FREE BREAKFAST HASH

SERVES (F) (M) 1   PREP : 5 MINUTES   COOK : 10 MINUTES

This is one of my most popular recipes. It's hard to believe we missed out on butter, bacon, chorizo and avocado for all those years when we were brainwashed to believe they would make us fat and give us heart disease. Although this recipe only serves one, trust me when I say it's worth making at least a double batch – it tastes just as good reheated the next day. Just make sure you add the avocado right before serving.

½ cup finely diced pumpkin
30g grass-fed butter
50g pasture-raised chorizo,
  finely diced
50g pasture-raised bacon,
  finely diced / 100g pasture-
  raised bacon, finely diced
½ zucchini, finely diced
½ cup finely chopped broccoli
1 cup spinach leaves
½ avocado, sliced /
  1 avocado, sliced
sea salt and pepper, to taste

1 Bring a small saucepan of water to the boil. Place pumpkin in a colander or steamer basket, cover with a lid and steam for 4–5 minutes.

2 Melt butter in a large frypan over medium heat and add pumpkin, chorizo and bacon. Cook until caramelised, stirring throughout.

4 Add zucchini and broccoli and sauté for 1–2 minutes, or until slightly softened. Add spinach and stir through well.

4 Remove from heat and transfer to a serving bowl. Top with avocado, season with salt and pepper, and enjoy.

(F) MACROS Cals : **721** CHO : **29g** P : **19g** Fat : **63g**
(M) MACROS Cals : **982** CHO : **34g** P : **22g** Fat : **92g**

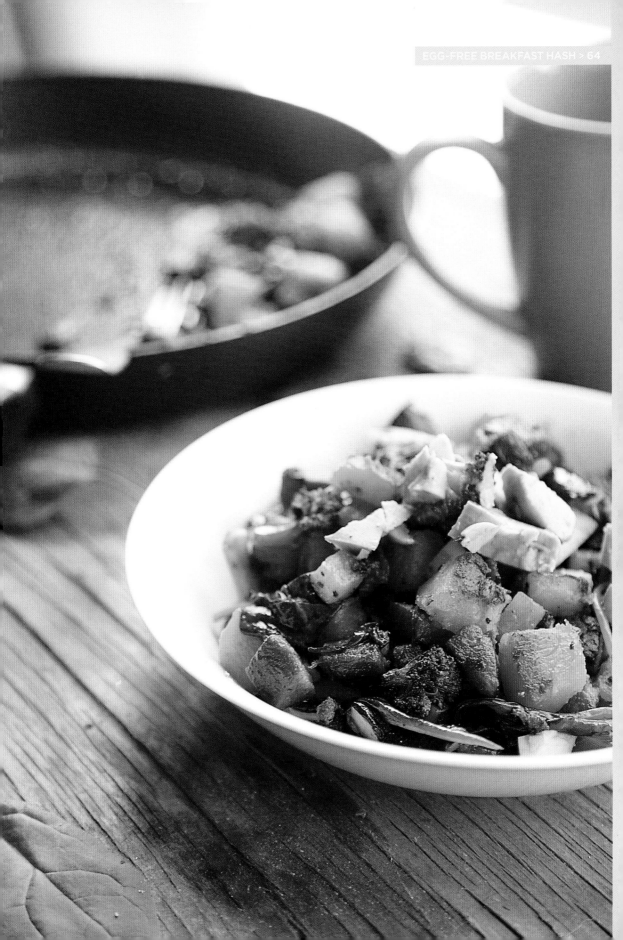

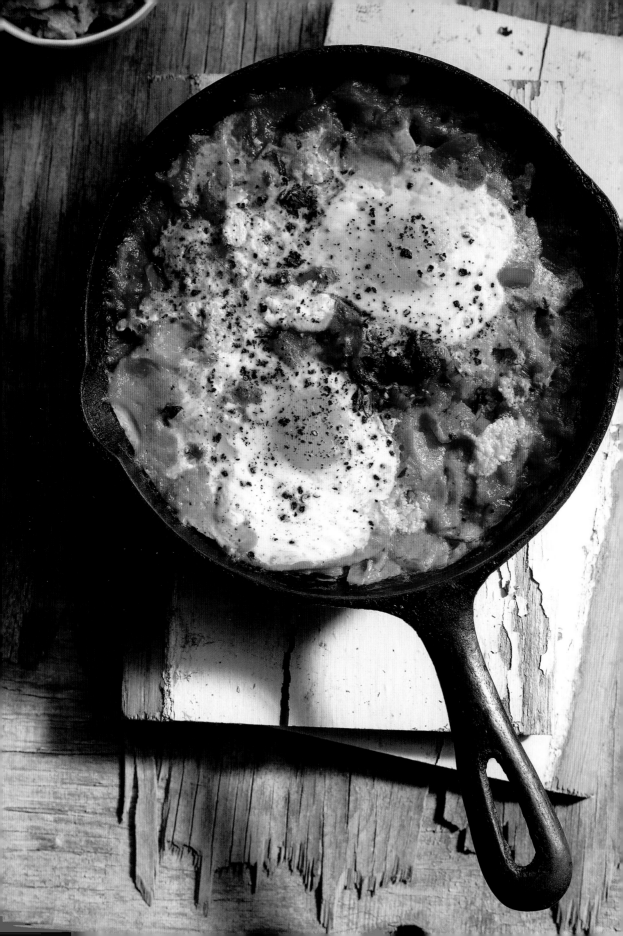

BASIC BAKED EGGS

SERVES Ⓕ♀ Ⓜ♂ 2 / 1   PREP : 15 MINUTES   COOK : 15 MINUTES

Baked eggs are such a delicious breakfast option, the whole family will enjoy them!
The addition of bone broth makes this a great gut-healing meal, and one that will
keep you satiated for hours.

100g leek, finely sliced
100g pasture-raised chorizo,
    diced
½ red capsicum, diced
½ teaspoon chilli flakes
400g can crushed tomatoes
¼ cup bone broth
20g spinach leaves, roughly
    chopped / 40g spinach
    leaves, roughly chopped
30g goat's feta
4 free-range eggs / 2 free-range
    eggs
sea salt and pepper, to taste
2 tablespoons chopped fresh
    parsley
1 avocado, mashed
1 slice of Almost Paleo Vegie
    Bread (see recipe page 206),
    for serving, optional

1   Preheat oven to 170°C.

2   Heat a large ovenproof frypan over medium heat and
    sauté leek, chorizo and capsicum for 3–4 minutes, or until
    softened. Add chilli flakes and continue to sauté for another
    minute.

3   Stir in tomatoes and bone broth and simmer for 6 minutes.
    Stir in spinach until wilted.

4   Dot the feta on top of the tomato mixture.

5   Make two or four holes in the mixture and crack an egg
    into each hole. Season with salt and pepper, and top with
    parsley.

6   Bake in the oven for 10–15 minutes, or until the eggs are
    cooked to your liking.

7   To serve, transfer to plates and top with mashed avocado,
    with toasted bread on the side, if you like.

Ⓕ♀ MACROS   Cals : 531   CHO : 21g   P : 29g   Fat : 37g
🍴   MACROS   Cals : 747   CHO : 32g   P : 38g   Fat : 53g
Ⓜ♂ MACROS   Cals : 829   CHO : 30g   P : 48g   Fat : 58g
🍴   MACROS   Cals : 1045 CHO : 41g   P : 57g   Fat : 74g

BREAKFAST SALAD WITH BOILED EGG

SERVES Ⓕ Ⓜ 1   PREP : 5 MINUTES   COOK : 15 MINUTES

I can't go past a good breakfast salad. My Almond Butter Dressing (see below) will definitely keep you coming back for more.

1 free-range egg / 2 free-range eggs
½ cup finely chopped broccoli
½ cup finely sliced kale (stalks removed)
1 teaspoon goji berries
½ cup spinach leaves
¼ bunch coriander, roughly chopped
¼ bunch basil, finely chopped
¼ cup almonds, roughly chopped
½ avocado, diced
sea salt and pepper, to taste

ALMOND BUTTER DRESSING
1 tablespoon almond butter
1 tablespoon extra-virgin olive oil / 2 tablespoons extra-virgin olive oil
1 lemon, zested and juiced

1   To boil egg/s: Bring a small saucepan of water to the boil. Carefully add eggs and reduce heat to a simmer. Cook for 4–5 minutes. Run under cold water before peeling and cutting in half.

2   Using the same saucepan, place broccoli in a colander or steamer basket, cover with a lid and steam for 4–5 minutes. Remove from the colander or steamer basket and set aside to cool.

3   To make the dressing, place the almond butter, olive oil, lemon zest and juice and 1 tablespoon of water in a small bowl and whisk until well combined. Whisk in a little extra water if a runnier dressing is required.

4   In a bowl, combine the kale and goji berries and half the dressing. Massage them for 1–2 minutes to soften.

5   Add spinach, broccoli, coriander, basil, almonds and avocado, and toss to combine. Season well with salt and pepper, top with boiled eggs and drizzle with extra dressing, if required. Store remaining dressing in the fridge for 5 days.

Egg-free variation: If you want to leave out the egg, add 2 tablespoons of pumpkin seeds in with the kale and goji berries instead.

Ⓕ MACROS Cals : **651** CHO : **26g** P : **23g** Fat : **56g**
Ⓜ MACROS Cals : **807** CHO : **26g** P : **26g** Fat : **69g**

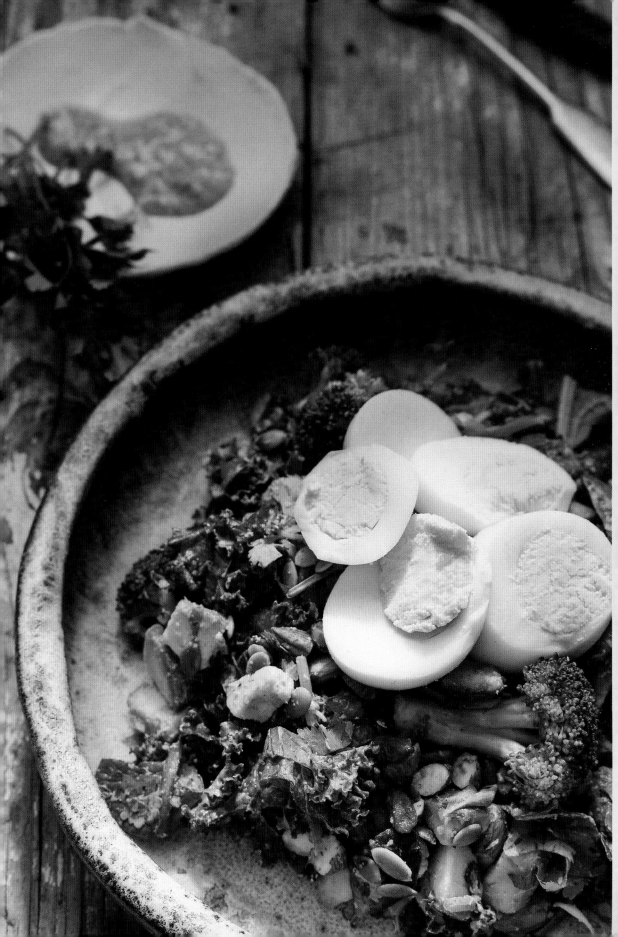

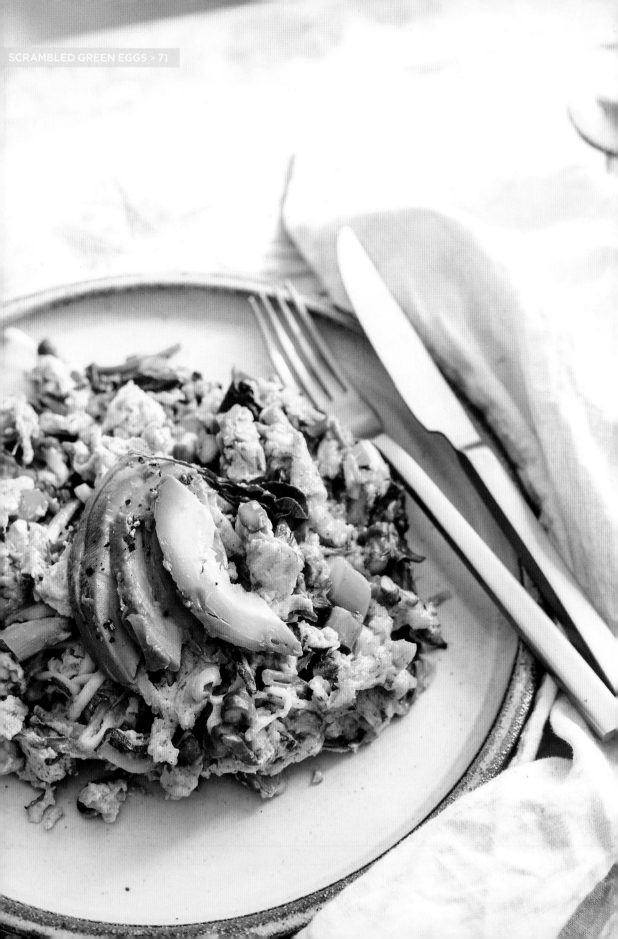

SCRAMBLED GREEN EGGS

SERVES (F) (M) 1   PREP : 10 MINUTES   COOK : 15 MINUTES

3 free-range eggs /
  4 free-range eggs
½ teaspoon turmeric
1 tablespoon cold-pressed
  extra-virgin coconut oil
½ bunch broccolini, roughly
  chopped
5 asparagus spears, roughly
  diced
1 zucchini, spiralised
20g spinach leaves, roughly
  chopped
sea salt and pepper, to taste
½ avocado, sliced /
  1 avocado, sliced

1   Whisk eggs and turmeric in a bowl until well combined.
    Set aside.

2   Heat a small frypan over medium heat and add oil,
    broccolini, asparagus and zucchini. Sauté until softened.
    Add spinach and continue to sauté until just starting to wilt.

3   Evenly pour in egg mixture and, using a wooden spoon or
    spatula, gently stir the egg around the greens. Continue
    doing this until the eggs are cooked to your liking. Season
    well with salt and pepper, and serve topped with sliced
    avocado.

(F) MACROS   Cals : **562**   CHO : **21g**   P : **26g**   Fat : **43g**

(M) MACROS   Cals : **716**   CHO : **25g**   P : **32g**   Fat : **43g**

SIMPLE BREAKFAST STIR-FRY

SERVES (F) (M) 2 / 1   PREP : 10 MINUTES   COOK : 15 MINUTES

A stir-fry for breakfast? With LCHF, gone are the days of recipes for specific meal
times – your body needs nutrients and your tastebuds really don't know what time it is!
The addition of sweet potato makes this an ideal post-training meal, but if you're not
training, simply balance out your overall carbohydrate load with subsequent lower-
carbohydrate meal choices.

½ sweet potato, diced
1 tablespoon cold-pressed
  extra-virgin coconut oil
¼ teaspoon cinnamon
sea salt and pepper, to taste
2 rashers pasture-raised
  bacon, diced
1 red capsicum, diced
4 stalks broccolini, roughly
  chopped
1 cup roughly chopped kale
4 free-range eggs / 2 free-range
  eggs
20g almonds, roughly chopped,
  optional

1   Preheat oven to 180°C and line a baking tray with baking
    paper.

2   Place diced sweet potato in a bowl and toss through half the
    oil and the cinnamon. Season well with salt and pepper and
    transfer to the baking tray. Bake for 15 minutes.

3   Heat remaining coconut oil in a frypan over medium heat
    and sauté bacon until golden. Add capsicum, broccolini and
    kale, and stir-fry quickly until softened. Toss through sweet
    potato then set aside.

4   In the same frypan, fry eggs to your liking. Serve the stir-fry
    vegetables topped with fried eggs. Scatter almonds on top,
    if using, and season again if required.

(F) MACROS   Cals : **577**   CHO : **21g**   P : **23g**   Fat : **46g**

(M) MACROS   Cals : **706**   CHO : **31g**   P : **37g**   Fat : **49g**

GREEN BAKED EGGS

SERVES (F) (M) 2 / 1   PREP : 10 MINUTES   COOK : 25 MINUTES

1 tablespoon cold-pressed
  extra-virgin coconut oil
100g pasture-raised chorizo, diced
1 leek, sliced
½ teaspoon garlic powder
1 green chilli, deseeded and
  finely chopped
1 teaspoon cumin
¼ cup bone broth
1 bunch asparagus, finely
  chopped
2 cups roughly chopped kale/
  1 cup roughly chopped kale
2 cups roughly chopped spinach
  leaves / 1 cup roughly
  chopped spinach leaves
60g goat's feta / 30g goat's feta
2 tablespoons pine nuts
1 tablespoon roughly chopped
  fresh parsley
4 free-range eggs / 2 free-range
  eggs
sea salt and pepper, to taste

1 Preheat oven to 170°C.

2 Heat a small ovenproof frypan over medium heat and add
   oil, chorizo, leek and garlic powder. Sauté for 3 minutes,
   or until chorizo and leek are golden.

3 Stir in chilli and cumin, add bone broth and simmer for
   4 minutes.

4 Stir in asparagus, kale and spinach and simmer until wilted.

5 Dot the mixture with feta, pine nuts and parsley.

6 Make two or four holes in the mixture and crack an egg into
   each hole. Season well with salt and pepper, and bake in the
   oven for 10–15 minutes, or until the eggs are cooked to your
   liking. Transfer to plates for serving.

(F) MACROS Cals : 583 CHO : 15g P : 34g Fat : 44g
(M) MACROS Cals : 831 CHO : 27g P : 48g Fat : 61g

CARROT CAKE CHIA PUDDING

SERVES (F) (M) 1   PREP : 5 MINUTES + OVERNIGHT SOAKING

3 tablespoons chia seeds /
  ¼ cup chia seeds
200ml coconut milk
1 teaspoon organic vanilla extract
½ cup grated carrot
1 tablespoon chopped walnuts /
  2 tablespoons chopped
  walnuts
¼ teaspoon cinnamon
¼ teaspoon sea salt

TO SERVE
50g coconut yoghurt /
  100g coconut yoghurt
1 teaspoon organic rice malt
  syrup, optional

1 Place all the pudding ingredients in an airtight container,
   stir thoroughly and soak overnight in the fridge. You may
   need to check on it once or twice and, stir again.

2 To serve, top with coconut yoghurt and, if you need a little
   more sweetness, rice malt syrup.

(F) MACROS Cals : 404 CHO : 24g P : 9g   Fat : 28g
(M) MACROS Cals : 600 CHO : 56g P : 22g Fat : 32g

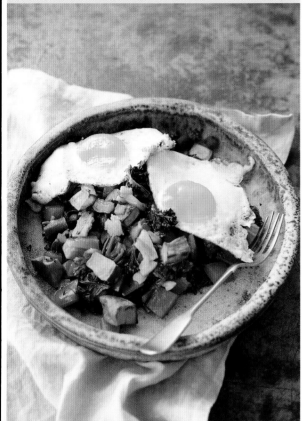

SIMPLE BREAKFAST STIR-FRY > 71

GREEN BAKED EGGS > 7

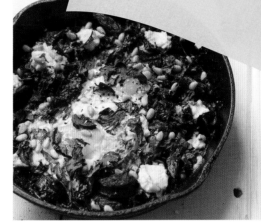

CARROT CAKE CHIA PUDDING > 72

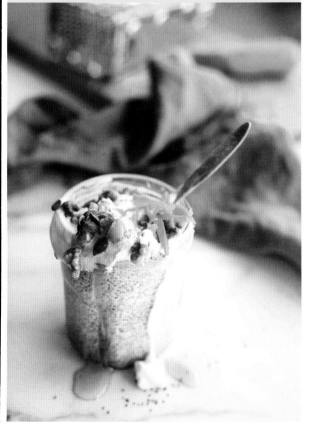

BREAKFAST STIR-FRY WITH TAHINI DRESSING > 75

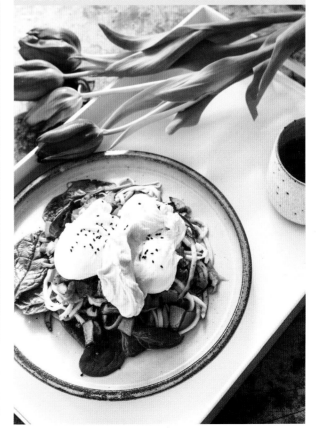

OATLESS OVERNIGHT PORRIDGE

SERVES (F)♀ (M)♂ 1   PREP : 10 MINUTES + OVERNIGHT SOAKING

Using quinoa instead of more traditional oats, this is an easy mid-week option for after exercise. The addition of LSA is great for digestive support, hormonal clearance and our magic 'S' word – satiety!

¼ banana
100ml coconut cream
2 tablespoons quinoa flakes
1 teaspoon unsweetened coconut flakes / 1 tablespoon unsweetened coconut flakes
1 tablespoon linseed, sunflower and almond meal (LSA)
30g grass-fed whey protein powder
1 tablespoon goji berries
1 teaspoon chia seeds
½ teaspoon organic vanilla extract

TO SERVE
1 tablespoon unsweetened coconut milk
¼ cup mixed berries

1 Place banana and coconut cream in a blender or food processor and blend until well combined.

2 Transfer to a bowl or glass jar and add remaining ingredients. Stir thoroughly to ensure all ingredients are well combined, cover and transfer to the fridge to soak overnight.

3 Before serving, stir through coconut milk and top with mixed berries.

(F)♀ MACROS Cals : **624** CHO : **47g** P : **39g** Fat : **32g**
(M)♂ MACROS Cals : **764** CHO : **61g** P : **41g** Fat : **42g**

BREAKFAST STIR-FRY WITH TAHINI DRESSING

SERVES Ⓕ Ⓜ 2   PREP : 10 MINUTES   COOK : 25 MINUTES

1 cup diced pumpkin
1 tablespoon cold-pressed
    extra-virgin coconut oil
¼ teaspoon cinnamon
sea salt and pepper
4 free-range eggs
dash of vinegar, for poaching
4 rashers pasture-raised
    bacon, diced
1 red capsicum, diced
6 asparagus spears, diced
2 zucchinis, spiralised
1 cup roughly chopped
    spinach leaves

TAHINI DRESSING
¼ cup tahini
1 lemon, zested and juiced
½ teaspoon garlic powder
½ teaspoon sea salt

1   Preheat oven to 180°C and line a baking tray with
    baking paper.

2   Place diced pumpkin in a bowl and toss with ½ tablespoon
    oil and the cinnamon. Season well with salt and pepper, and
    transfer to the baking tray. Bake for 15 minutes.

3   To poach eggs: Bring a small saucepan of water to the boil.
    Add a dash of vinegar. Crack an egg into a cup and create
    a gentle whirlpool in the water. Slowly tip the egg into the
    water, white first, and leave to cook for 3 minutes. Remove
    with a slotted spoon and drain on paper towel. Repeat for
    each additional egg.

4   Meanwhile, heat remaining oil in a frypan over medium heat
    and sauté bacon until golden. Add capsicum and asparagus
    and stir-fry for 4 minutes. Add zucchini noodles and spinach
    and stir-fry quickly until softened. Toss through pumpkin.

5   To make the dressing, combine all the ingredients plus
    1 tablespoon of water in a glass jar and whisk well to
    combine. Whisk in a little extra water if you would like a
    thinner consistency.

6   Divide vegetable mixture between two plates, top with
    poached eggs and drizzle with tahini dressing. Store any
    remaining dressing in the fridge for 5 days.

Ⓕ MACROS Cals : **498** CHO : **31g** P : **35g** Fat : **71g**
Ⓜ MACROS Cals : **498** CHO : **31g** P : **35g** Fat : **71g**

LSA & CHIA PUDDING WITH RASPBERRIES > 77

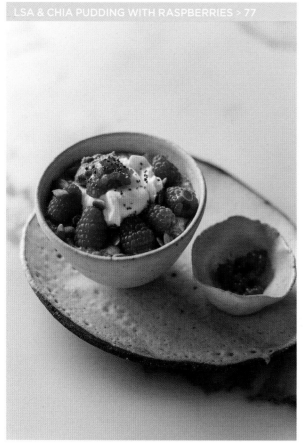

LSA 'PORRIDGE' > 77

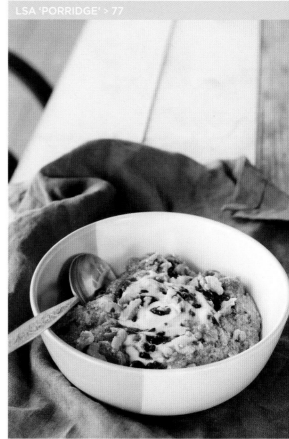

OATLESS OVERNIGHT PORRIDGE > 74

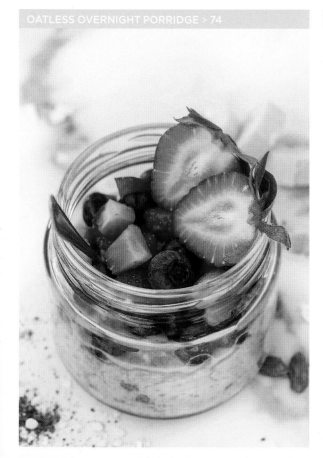

GLUTEN-FREE AND SUGAR-FREE GRANOLA > 79

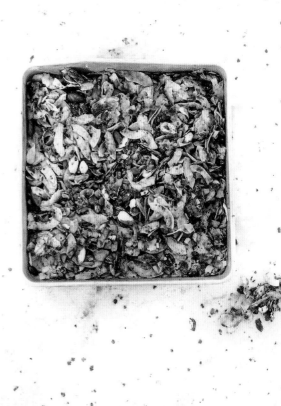

LSA & CHIA PUDDING WITH RASPBERRIES

SERVES Ⓕ Ⓜ 1   PREP : 5 MINUTES + OVERNIGHT SOAKING

2 tablespoons linseed, sunflower
and almond meal (LSA) /
3 tablespoons linseed,
sunflower and almond meal
(LSA)
½ tablespoon chia seeds /
1 tablespoon chia seeds
¼ teaspoon organic rice malt
syrup / ½ teaspoon organic
rice malt syrup
150ml coconut milk /
200ml coconut milk

TO SERVE
½ cup raspberries /
1 cup raspberries
½ **lemon, zested**
1 tablespoon coconut yoghurt /
¼ cup coconut yoghurt
1 teaspoon pumpkin seeds /
1 tablespoon pumpkin seeds
1 teaspoon almond butter /
1 tablespoon almond butter

1 Place all the pudding ingredients in an airtight container,
stir thoroughly and soak overnight in the fridge. You may
need to check on it once or twice and, stir again.

2 Before serving, combine raspberries with lemon zest
in a bowl and roughly mash. Set aside.

3 To serve, top the pudding with the raspberry mixture,
coconut yoghurt, pumpkin seeds and almond butter.

Ⓕ MACROS Cals : **459** CHO : **38g** P : **17g** Fat : **34g**
Ⓜ MACROS Cals : **669** CHO : **48g** P : **22g** Fat : **51g**

LCHF 'PORRIDGE'

SERVES Ⓕ Ⓜ 1   PREP : 10 MINUTES   COOK : 15 MINUTES

My LCHF porridge uses cauliflower instead of oats or quinoa. Try it, you will be
pleasantly surprised. It's a great one to batch-cook for the entire week. Replace the
rice malt syrup with stevia if you need to lower your carbs further.

1 cup cauliflower rice (approx.
¼ head of cauliflower, chopped)
1 cup unsweetened coconut milk
1 tablespoon almond butter /
2 tablespoons almond butter
1 tablespoon shredded coconut /
2 tablespoons shredded
coconut
1 teaspoon organic rice malt syrup
½ teaspoon cinnamon
¼ teaspoon organic vanilla extract
¼ teaspoon sea salt
½ cup raspberries, for serving

1 To make the cauliflower rice: Place chopped cauliflower in
a food processor or blender and blitz until it resembles rice.

2 Place the cauliflower rice and all the remaining ingredients,
except for raspberries, in a small saucepan over medium
heat. Cook, stirring regularly, for 10 minutes, or until
cauliflower is tender and liquid absorbed. Increase heat
to high for a further 5 minutes, making sure you continue
stirring so it does not overboil.

3 Remove from heat, stir in raspberries and serve.

Ⓕ MACROS Cals : **398** CHO : **44g** P : **7g** Fat : **23g**
Ⓜ MACROS Cals : **547** CHO : **46g** P : **9g** Fat : **39g**

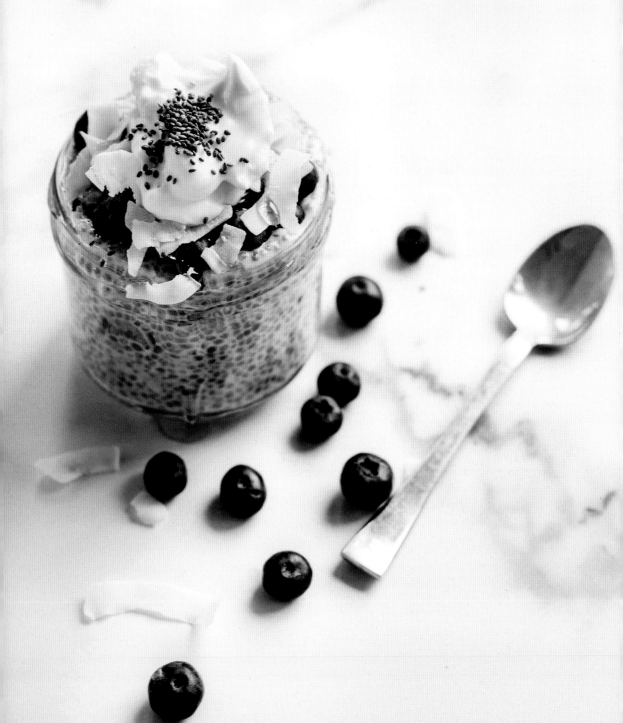

GLUTEN-FREE & SUGAR-FREE GRANOLA

SERVES (F) (M) 10   PREP : 5 MINUTES   COOK : 10 MINUTES

For most people, finding a breakfast replacement for their conventional cereal can be one of the first LCHF hurdles they face. This granola is the answer you have been looking for – the only challenge now will be your portion control, it's that good!

2 cups unsweetened coconut flakes
1 cup raw almonds, chopped
¼ cup pumpkin seeds
¼ cup sunflower seeds
2 tablespoons chia seeds
1 tablespoon cinnamon
¼ cup cold-pressed extra-virgin coconut oil
2 tablespoons organic rice malt syrup

TO SERVE, PER PERSON
100g coconut yoghurt /
    150g coconut yoghurt
½ cup raspberries

1   Preheat oven to 180°C and line a baking tray with baking paper.
2   Place all the ingredients in a large bowl and mix thoroughly.
3   Spread evenly on the baking tray and place in the oven for 10–15 minutes, checking and stirring regularly.
4   Remove from the oven and allow to cool.
5   Transfer to an airtight container and keep in the fridge for extra crunch.
6   Serve with coconut yoghurt and raspberries.

(F) MACROS   Cals : **514**   CHO : **29g**   P : **19g**   Fat : **63g**
(M) MACROS   Cals : **819**   CHO : **57g**   P : **22g**   Fat : **63g**

BERRY & COCONUT CHIA PUDDING

SERVES (F) (M) 1   PREP : 5 MINUTES + OVERNIGHT SOAKING

Chia puddings are another great mid-week breakfast. While they don't necessarily contain vegetables, they are a far better option than conventional cereal or toast. To fast-track your morning, prepare the puddings on Sunday or the night before. They will last two or three days in the fridge.

3 tablespoons chia seeds
250ml unsweetened almond milk
1 teaspoon organic rice malt syrup
1 teaspoon organic vanilla extract
30g almonds, chopped
½ cup blueberries

TO SERVE
1 tablespoon coconut yoghurt /
    ¼ cup coconut yoghurt
1 teaspoon unsweetened coconut flakes
1 tablespoon almond butter, optional

1   Place all the pudding ingredients in an airtight container, stir thoroughly and soak overnight in the fridge. You may need to check on it once or twice and, stir again.
2   To serve, top with remaining blueberries, yoghurt, coconut flakes and almond butter, if using.

(F) MACROS   Cals : **425**   CHO : **38g**   P : **10g**   Fat : **27g**
(M) MACROS   Cals : **658**   CHO : **35g**   P : **20g**   Fat : **51g**

BAKED ZUCCHINI PANCAKES

SERVES Ⓕ Ⓜ 1   PREP : 15 MINUTES   COOK : 20 MINUTES

These taste even better than they look! This is one of my favourite breakfasts to make on a Sunday, and they double as a delicious lunch.

½ tablespoon cold-pressed extra-virgin coconut oil, melted + ½ tablespoon extra
2 tablespoons chia seeds
½ zucchini, roughly chopped
2 tablespoons almond flour
2 tablespoons coconut flour
1 teaspoon gluten-free baking powder
1 teaspoon tapioca
½ teaspoon psyllium husks
½ teaspoon sea salt

AVOCADO MASH

¼ avocado / ½ avocado
100g cherry tomatoes, roughly chopped
20g rocket leaves
1 teaspoon lemon juice
sea salt and pepper, to taste

1 Preheat oven to 180°C and line a baking tray with baking paper. Melt ½ tablespoon coconut oil and set aside.

2 Prepare the 'chia seed eggs' in a bowl by combining chia seeds with 120ml water. Stir well and rest for 15 minutes.

3 In a food processor or blender, place all the pancake ingredients, including the 'chia seed eggs' and the remaining coconut oil. Blend until well combined.

4 Divide mixture into three mounds on the prepared baking tray. Using the back of a spoon, spread the mixture into the shape and size you desire.

5 Bake in the oven for 15–20 minutes, or until golden brown. Flip at the halfway mark.

6 While the pancakes are cooking, place avocado, cherry tomatoes, rocket and lemon juice in a bowl. Mash roughly, and season well with salt and pepper.

7 To serve, stack pancakes on a plate and top with the avocado mash.

Ⓕ MACROS Cals : **486** CHO : **31g** P : **14g** Fat : **35g**
Ⓜ MACROS Cals : **545** CHO : **34g** P : **14g** Fat : **40g**

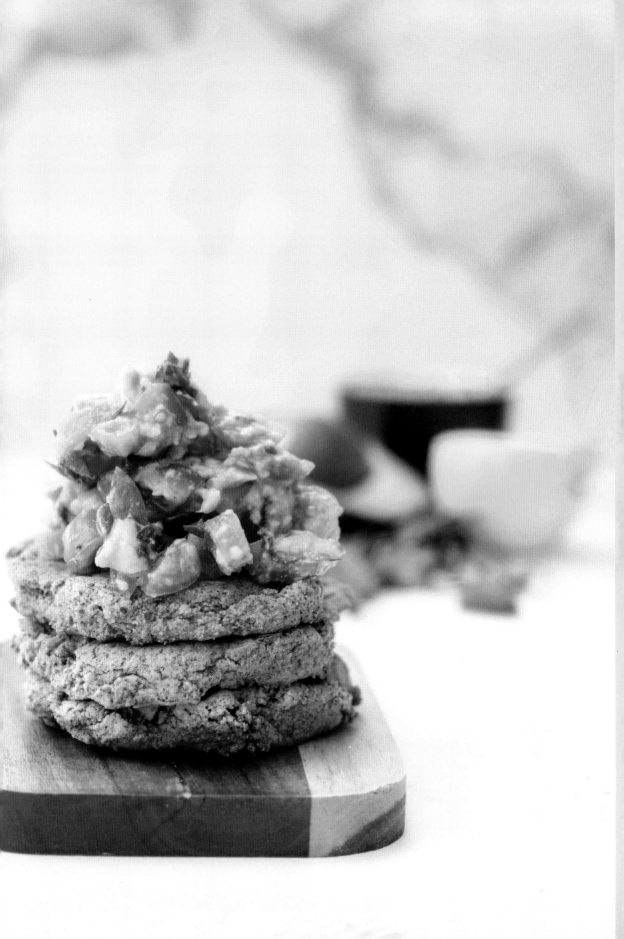

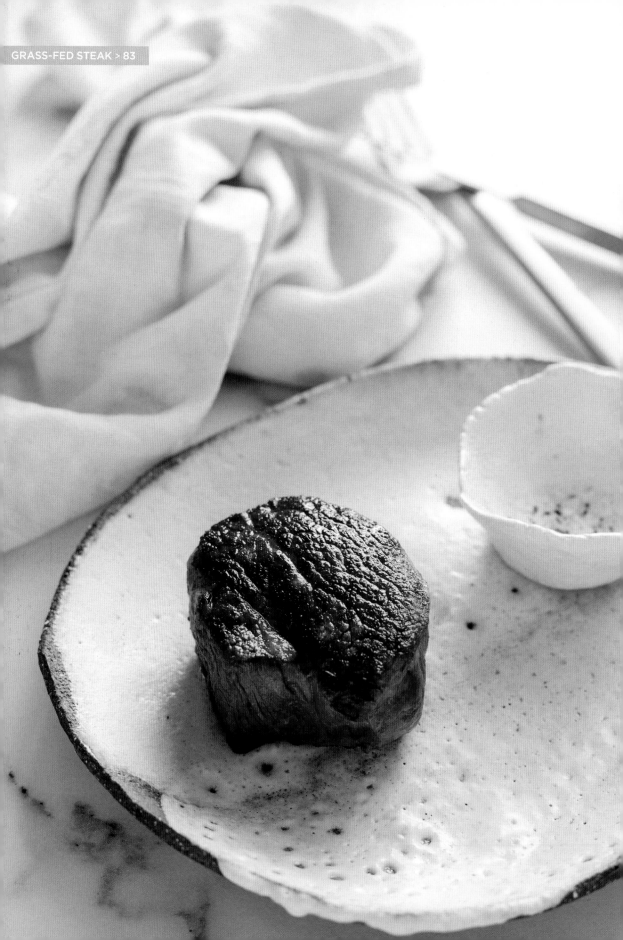

Eating the LCHF way can be simple and delicious. If you are short on time, I encourage you to pick one of the following simple proteins and pair it with your choice of salad or side dish for the perfect nutrient-dense dinner.

GRASS-FED STEAK

SERVES Ⓕ Ⓜ 2   PREP : 5 MINUTES + 1–2 HOURS MARINATING   COOK : 10 MINUTES

2 × 120g grass-fed beef eye fillets / 2 × 150g grass-fed beef eye fillets

2 tablespoons extra-virgin olive oil / 4 tablespoons extra-virgin olive oil

sea salt and pepper, to taste

1 Marinate steak in olive oil, sea salt and pepper for 1–2 hours.

2 Drain marinade into a preheated frypan over medium–high heat before adding steak and cooking for 6–8 minutes per side, depending on your desired result. Rest for 5 minutes before serving.

Ⓕ MACROS   Cals : **263**   CHO : **1g**   P : **25g**   Fat : **18g**
Ⓜ MACROS   Cals : **413**   CHO : **2g**   P : **32g**   Fat : **33g**

GLUTEN-FREE CHICKEN SCHNITZ

SERVES Ⓕ Ⓜ 4   PREP : 10 MINUTES   COOK : 10 MINUTES

This is another extremely popular and family-friendly recipe. Pair with your choice of a side, such as Buttered Greens or Simple Tomato Salad (see recipes pages 192 and 201).

1 free-range egg
1 cup almond meal
2 lemons (1 zested, 1 quartered)
sea salt and pepper, to taste
500g free-range chicken breast fillets, sliced in half widthways / 600g free-range chicken breast fillets, sliced in half widthways
2 tablespoons cold-pressed extra-virgin coconut oil
2 tablespoons chopped fresh parsley

1 In a small bowl, beat the egg. In a separate bowl, combine almond meal and the zest of 1 lemon, and season well with salt and pepper.

2 Lightly coat each chicken piece in the egg followed by the almond mix.

3 Heat coconut oil in a frypan over low–medium heat, add the chicken and cook for 5 minutes on each side, or until lightly golden.

4 Sprinkle chicken with chopped parsley and serve with a lemon wedge.

Ⓕ MACROS   Cals : **414**   CHO : **7g**   P : **36g**   Fat : **27g**
Ⓜ MACROS   Cals : **434**   CHO : **7g**   P : **40g**   Fat : **27g**

LAMB CUTLETS

SERVES Ⓕ Ⓜ 2   PREP : 5 MINUTES + 1–2 HOURS MARINATING   COOK : 10 MINUTES

6 grass-fed lamb cutlets /
  8 grass-fed lamb cutlets
¼ cup extra-virgin olive oil
sea salt and pepper, to taste

1 Marinate lamb cutlets in oil, sea salt and pepper for 1–2 hours.

2 Drain marinade into a preheated frypan over medium–high heat before adding cutlets and cooking for 4–6 minutes per side, or until cooked to your liking. Rest for 5 minutes before serving.

Ⓕ MACROS Cals : **405** CHO : **0g**   P : **26g** Fat : **36g**
Ⓜ MACROS Cals : **460** CHO : **0g**   P : **34g** Fat : **38g**

CLEAN CHICKEN PARMA

SERVES Ⓕ Ⓜ 4   PREP : 10 MINUTES   COOK : 15 MINUTES

1 free-range egg
1 cup almond or hazelnut meal
1 tablespoon coconut flour
sea salt and pepper, to taste
400g free-range chicken thigh
  fillets / 600g free-range
  chicken thigh fillets
½ cup cold-pressed extra-virgin
  coconut oil
4 slices ham, free range
Sugar-free Tomato Sauce (see
  recipe page 205)
2 slices organic hard cheese

1 Preheat oven to 180°C and line a baking tray with baking paper.

2 Place egg in a small bowl and whisk well. In a separate bowl, combine almond or hazelnut meal and coconut flour and season.

3 Cover chicken thighs well in egg, then coat well in the flour mix.

4 Heat coconut oil in a large frypan over medium–high heat and shallow-fry chicken for 5 minutes per side, or until lightly browned.

5 Transfer onto the lined baking tray. Place ham on top of chicken, add 1–2 tablespoons of Sugar-free Tomato Sauce and top with cheese.

6 Bake in the oven for 5 minutes or until cheese has melted.

Ⓕ MACROS Cals : **644** CHO : **7g**   P : **39g** Fat : **45g**
Ⓜ MACROS Cals : **701** CHO : **7g**   P : **49g** Fat : **47g**

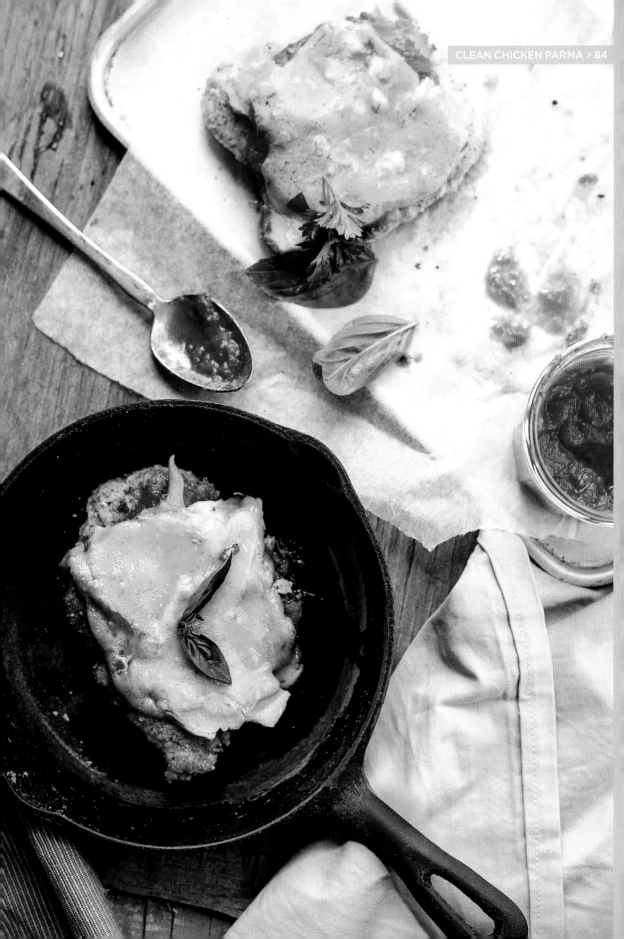

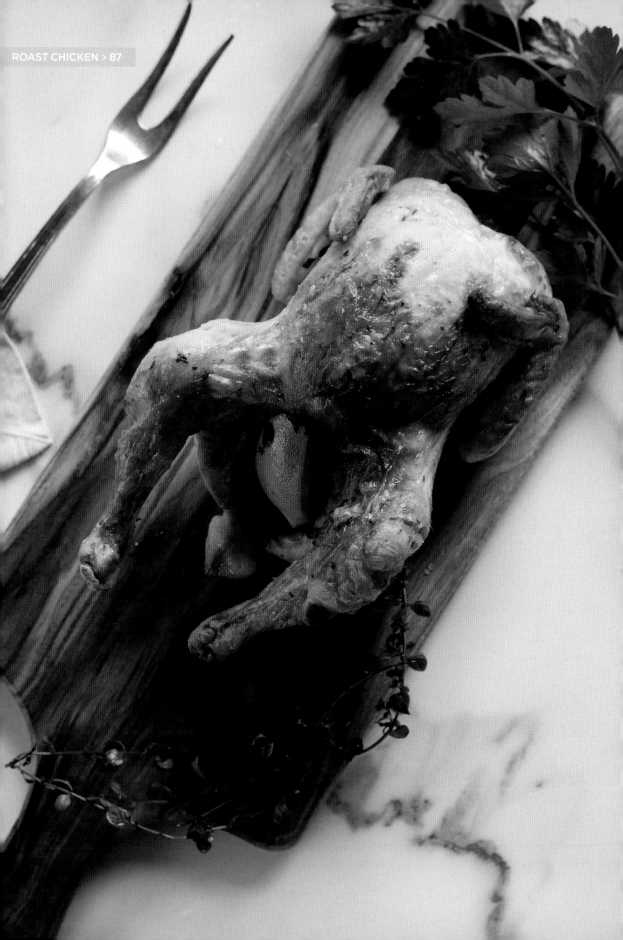

ROAST CHICKEN

SERVES (F)(M) 6 / 4   PREP : 5 MINUTES   COOK : 1¼ HOURS

1 whole free-range chicken, approximately 1.8kg
1 lemon, halved
2 tablespoons roughly chopped fresh parsley
2 tablespoons fresh thyme leaves
sea salt and pepper, to taste
2 tablespoons extra-virgin olive oil

1 Preheat oven to 180°C and line a roasting tray with baking paper.
2 Stuff the chicken with lemon and herbs, and season generously with salt and pepper. Score the drumsticks with a paring knife and rub olive oil over entire chicken.
3 Place the chicken on the roasting tray and roast for 1¼ hours, or until crispy and golden brown on the outside and the juices run clear. Rest for 10 minutes before serving.
4 Alternatively, have your butcher butterfly the chicken. Place the chicken flat on the roasting tray. Score the drumsticks with a paring knife. Season chicken generously with herbs, salt, pepper and olive oil. Roast for 45 minutes, or until crispy and golden brown on the outside and the juices run clear. Rest for 10 minutes before serving.

(F) MACROS Cals : 211 CHO : 0g P : 20g Fat : 15g
(M) MACROS Cals : 317 CHO : 0g P : 30g Fat : 22g

PORK CUTLETS

SERVES (F)(M) 2   PREP : 5 MINUTES + 1–2 HOURS MARINATING   COOK : 10 MINUTES

2 × 120g pork cutlets /
2 × 150g pork cutlets
1 tablespoon extra-virgin olive oil
1 teaspoon dried sage or chilli flakes
¼ teaspoon sea salt

1 Marinate pork cutlets in oil, sage or chilli flakes and sea salt for 1–2 hours.
2 Drain marinade into a preheated frypan over medium–high heat before adding cutlets and cooking for 6–8 minutes per side, or until cooked to your liking. Rest for 5 minutes before serving.

(F) MACROS Cals : 414 CHO : 0g P : 24g Fat : 27g
(M) MACROS Cals : 503 CHO : 0g P : 30g Fat : 32g

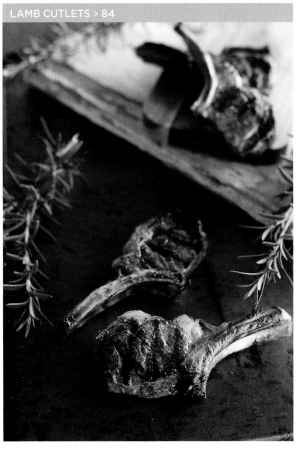

LAMB CUTLETS > 84

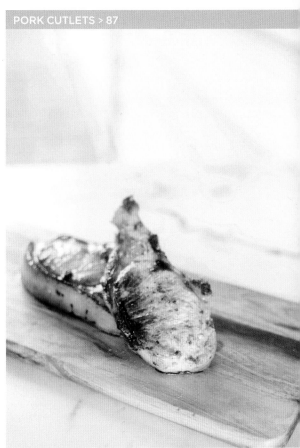

PORK CUTLETS > 87

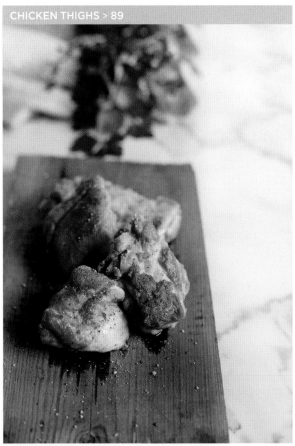

CHICKEN THIGHS > 89

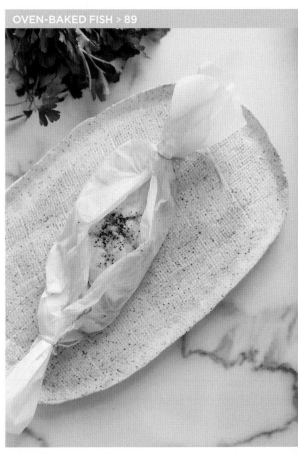

OVEN-BAKED FISH > 89

CHICKEN THIGHS

SERVES (F)(M) 2   PREP : 5 MINUTES + 1–2 HOURS MARINATING   COOK : 10 MINUTES

240g free-range chicken thigh
  fillet / 300g free-range
  chicken thigh fillet
¼ cup extra-virgin olive oil
sea salt and pepper, to taste

1 Marinate chicken in oil, sea salt and pepper for 1–2 hours.
2 Drain marinade into a preheated frypan over medium heat before adding chicken and cooking for 10 minutes per side, or until golden and cooked through. Rest for 5 minutes before serving.

(F) MACROS Cals : **409** CHO : **0g** P : **23g** Fat : **36g**
(M) MACROS Cals : **452** CHO : **0g** P : **29g** Fat : **39g**

OVEN-BAKED FISH

SERVES (F)(M) 2   PREP : 5 MINUTES   COOK : 15 MINUTES

2 × 120g fillets of firm white fish
  such as barramundi / 2 × 175g
  fillets of firm white fish such
  as barramundi
2 tablespoons extra-virgin
  olive oil
sea salt and pepper, to taste
1 lemon, sliced

1 Preheat oven to 200°C.
2 Take two pieces of foil, large enough to wrap each fish fillet, and line each with a square of baking paper.
3 Place the fish, skin side down, on the baking paper. Drizzle with oil and season well with salt and pepper. Place 2–4 slices of lemon on top of each piece of fish. Wrap the fish in foil to form a parcel, sealing the edges by folding over the foil, and place on a baking tray. Bake for 10–15 minutes. Check the fish and if not cooked to your liking, simply re-seal the foil and place back in the oven for a few extra minutes.

(F) MACROS Cals : **222** CHO : **0g** P : **23g** Fat : **15g**
(M) MACROS Cals : **273** CHO : **0g** P : **34g** Fat : **15g**

SALMON FILLET

SERVES (F)(M) 2   PREP : 10 MINUTES   COOK : 10 MINUTES

1 tablespoon cold-pressed
  extra-virgin coconut oil
2 × 120g salmon fillets,
  preferably wild caught /
  2 × 150g salmon fillets,
  preferably wild caught
sea salt and pepper, to taste

1 Heat coconut oil in a frypan over medium–high heat and add salmon fillets, skin side down. Season with salt and pepper and cook for 5 minutes, or until skin is crispy, then flip the salmon and continue cooking the other side to your liking.

(F) MACROS Cals : **223** CHO : **0g** P : **23g** Fat : **14g**
(M) MACROS Cals : **264** CHO : **0g** P : **29g** Fat : **16g**

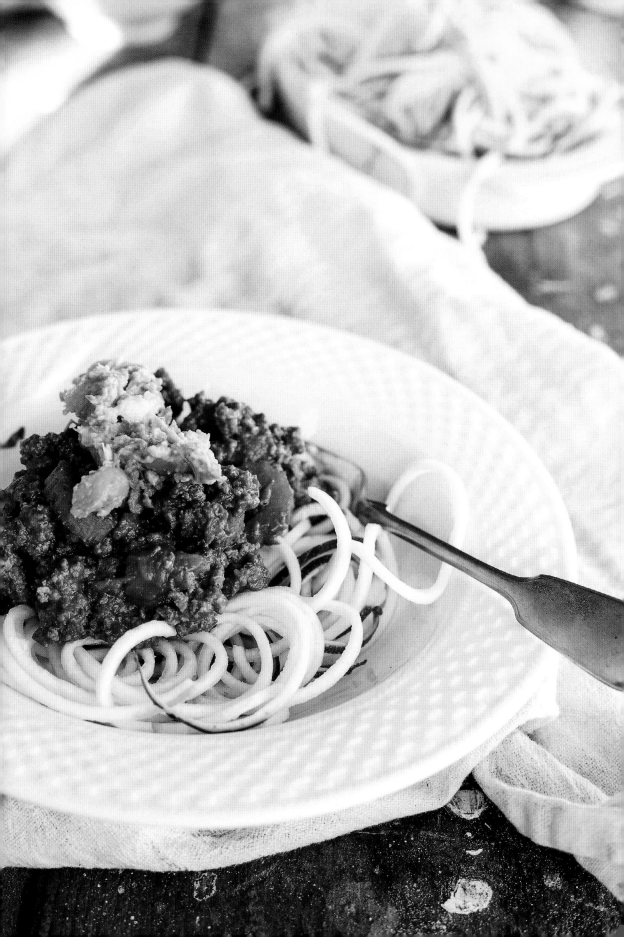

MAINS

Here's a collection of my favourite LCHF mains that I'm confident your loved ones will also enjoy. These recipes offer simplicity and variety and will transform many of your favourite recipes into lower carbohydrates versions. I promise you won't miss pasta, rice or burgers eating the LCHF way!

ZUCCHINI 'SPAGHETTI' BOLOGNESE

SERVES Ⓕ Ⓜ 4   PREP : 10 MINUTES   COOK : 30 MINUTES

I've been using zucchini instead of pasta for years now. It's such a great way to make a traditionally high-carb meal very LCHF friendly. My Zucchini Spaghetti Bolognese is great to batch-cook for a busy week ahead, and the sauce freezes really well.

1 tablespoon cold-pressed extra-virgin coconut oil
2 garlic cloves, finely chopped
500g grass-fed beef mince / 600g grass-fed beef mince
400g tomato passata (100% tomatoes)
2 tablespoons tomato paste (no salt added)
1 teaspoon chilli flakes
1 carrot
4 zucchinis
1 tablespoon grass-fed butter
1 cup grated organic hard cheese / 2 cups grated organic hard cheese
sea salt and pepper, to taste

1   Heat coconut oil in a large frypan over medium heat and lightly brown the garlic.

2   Add beef mince and cook until brown, stirring to remove any lumps.

3   Stir in tomato passata, tomato paste and chilli flakes. Simmer until most of the liquid has evaporated. Set aside.

4   Grate carrot and stir through the mince mixture.

5   Spiralise or slice zucchini to your desired thickness to make 'spaghetti', and sauté in a saucepan with the butter (or serve raw if you prefer).

6   Place zucchini 'spaghetti' in a bowl, top with bolognese sauce and grated cheese. Season well with salt and pepper.

Ⓕ MACROS Cals : 478   CHO : 13g   P : 34g   Fat : 33g
Ⓜ MACROS Cals : 640   CHO : 13g   P : 46g   Fat : 49g

CHILLI CON CARNE WITH AVOCADO SMASH

SERVES Ⓕ Ⓜ 4 / 2   PREP : 10 MINUTES   COOK : 15 MINUTES

1 tablespoon cold-pressed
  extra-virgin coconut oil
3 garlic cloves, crushed
1 red onion, diced
1 large red chilli, deseeded and
  finely chopped
2 red capsicums, diced
2 × 400g cans red kidney beans
400g can whole tomatoes
1 tablespoon tomato paste
  (no salt added)
1 bay leaf
3 teaspoons cumin
1 cup finely chopped kale
  leaves (stalks removed)
sea salt and pepper, to taste

AVOCADO SMASH
2 avocados, diced
½ cup coriander leaves,
  finely chopped
½ lime, juiced
2 tablespoons extra-virgin
  olive oil

1 Heat oil in a large frypan over medium heat. Add garlic,
   onion, chilli and capsicum, and sauté for 2–3 minutes,
   or until softened.

2 Add kidney beans, tomatoes, tomato paste, bay leaf, cumin,
   kale and ¼ cup of water to the pan, stir to combine then
   simmer for 10 minutes. Season well with salt and pepper.

3 Meanwhile, dice avocados and place in a bowl with the
   coriander, lime juice and olive oil. Roughly crush the
   ingredients with the back of a fork.

4 Serve the chilli con carne topped with smashed avocado.

Ⓕ MACROS Cals : **386** CHO : **31g**   P : **14g**   Fat : **22g**
Ⓜ MACROS Cals : **771** CHO : **61g**   P : **29g**   Fat : **45g**

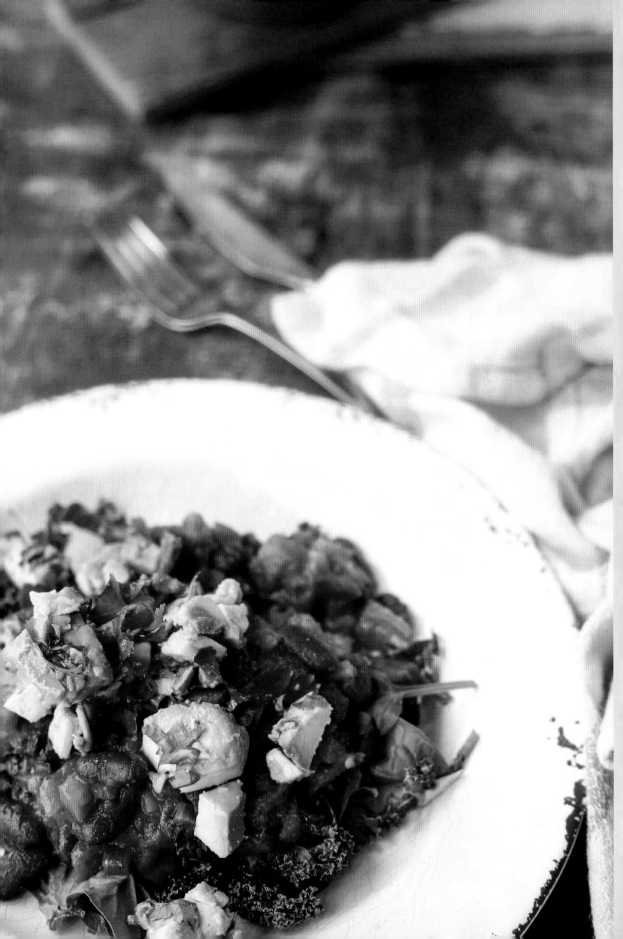

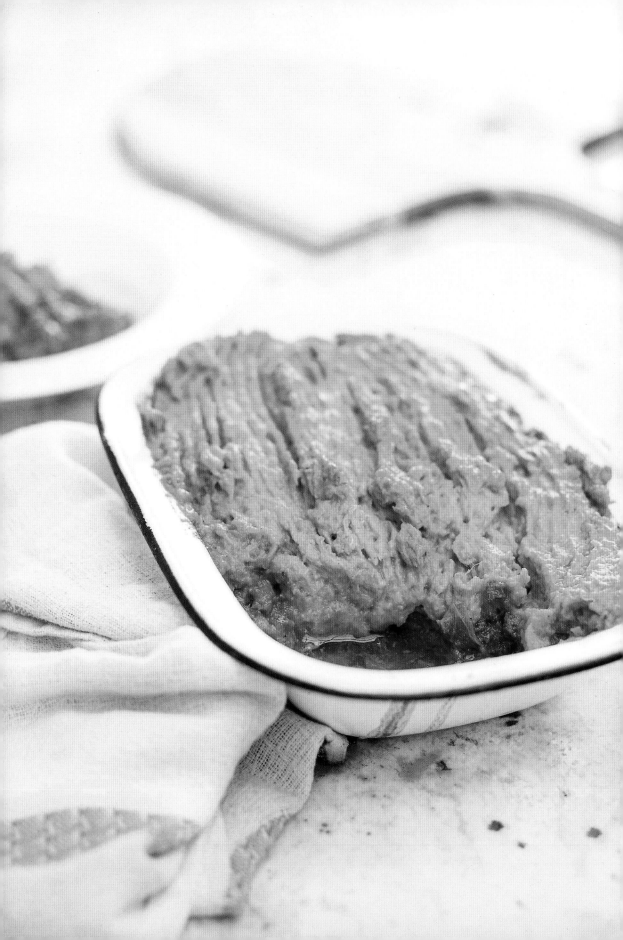

SHEPHERD'S PIE WITH PUMPKIN MASH

SERVES Ⓕ Ⓜ 6 / 4   PREP : 20 MINUTES   COOK : 20 MINUTES

This is another one of my weekly staple recipes. Pumpkin, although similar in colour to sweet potato, is surprisingly less starchy but just as delicious. The Pumpkin Mash recipe is on page 114.

1 tablespoon cold-pressed extra-virgin coconut oil
2 garlic cloves, chopped
500g grass-fed beef mince / 600g grass-fed beef mince
400g tomato passata (100% tomatoes)
2 tablespoons tomato paste (no salt added)
1 teaspoon chilli flakes
1 teaspoon cinnamon
1 teaspoon nutmeg
sea salt and pepper, to taste
1 carrot, grated
1 zucchini, grated

1   Preheat the oven to 220°C.

2   Heat oil in a large frypan over medium heat and sauté garlic until golden brown.

3   Add mince and cook for 15 minutes, stirring to remove any lumps.

4   Stir in tomato passata, tomato paste and spices, season and cook over low heat until the excess liquid evaporates.

5   While the mince mixture is cooking, make the Pumpkin Mash (see recipe page 114).

6   Stir the grated carrot and zucchini into the mince mixture and transfer to an 18cm baking dish, spreading until level.

7   Gently spoon the pumpkin mash over the top and press firmly until even.

8   Bake for 20 minutes, then finish under the grill so the top is crispy and brown. Serve with a side of salad, such as my Simple Tomato Salad (see recipe page 201).

Ⓕ   MACROS   Cals : **350**   CHO : **15g**   P : **30g**   Fat : **18g**
Ⓜ   MACROS   Cals : **512**   CHO : **20g**   P : **32g**   Fat : **35g**

SAVOURY MINCE WITH AVOCADO & STEAMED BROCCOLI

SERVES Ⓕ Ⓜ 4   PREP : 10 MINUTES   COOK : 20 MINUTES

1 tablespoon cold-pressed
  extra-virgin coconut oil
½ onion, finely chopped /
  1 onion, finely chopped
1 garlic clove, crushed
1 red capsicum, diced
½ teaspoon chilli flakes
1 teaspoon paprika
500g grass-fed beef mince
400g can chopped tomatoes
¼ cup bone broth
40g spinach leaves /
  60g spinach leaves
sea salt and pepper, to taste
¼ bunch parsley, chopped

TO SERVE
1 head of broccoli, cut into florets
1 avocado, mashed /
  2 avocados, mashed
1 tablespoon extra-virgin olive
  oil / 2 tablespoons extra-virgin
  olive oil

1　In a large frypan, melt coconut oil over medium heat and stir-fry onion, garlic, capsicum, chilli flakes and paprika until golden.

2　Add beef mince and cook until brown, stirring to remove any lumps.

3　Stir in chopped tomatoes and bone broth and simmer over low heat for 15 minutes.

4　Add spinach and continue to simmer until wilted. Season well with salt and pepper and stir through parsley.

5　While the mince is simmering, bring a small saucepan of water to the boil. Place broccoli in a colander or steamer basket, cover with a lid and steam for 4–5 minutes.

6　Serve the mince with the broccoli, top with mashed avocado and drizzle with olive oil.

Ⓕ MACROS Cals : **416**   CHO : **12g**   P : **29g** Fat : **29g**
Ⓜ MACROS Cals : **513**   CHO : **16g**   P : **30g** Fat : **38g**

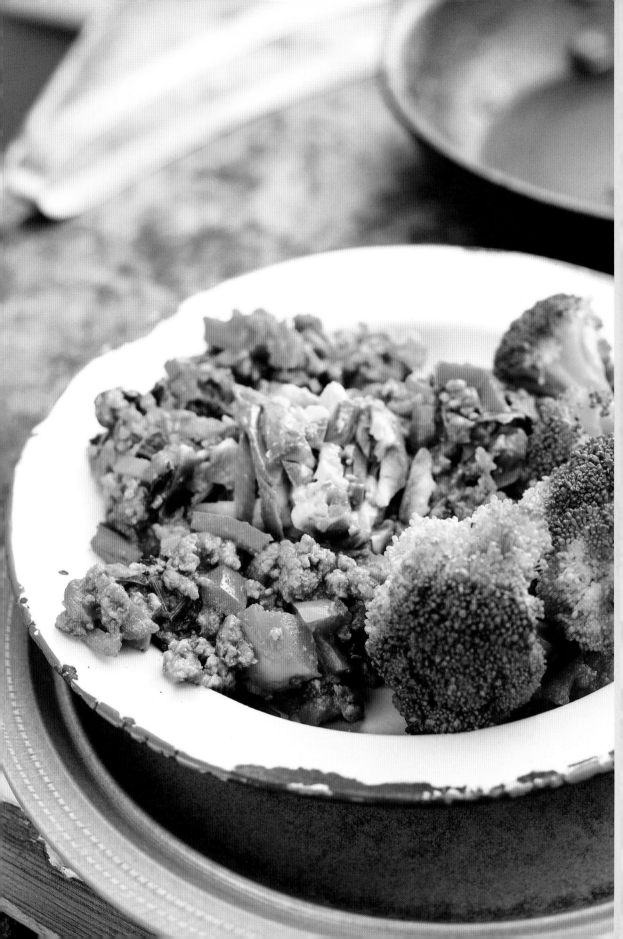

STEAK WITH WARM BROCCOLI SALAD > 99

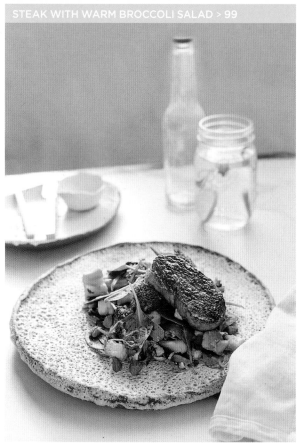

STEAK WITH ZUCCHINI & BRUSSELS SPROUTS > 100

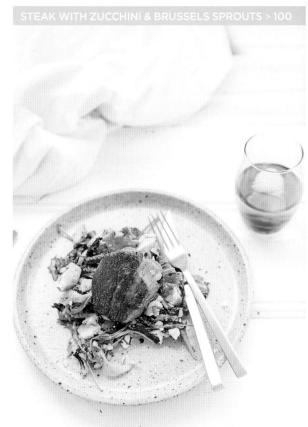

STEAK WITH BEETROOT & ORANGE SALAD > 100

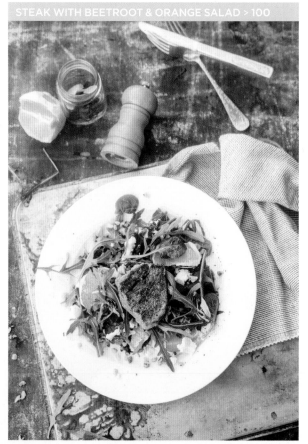

STEAK WITH ROCKET, WALNUT & PEAR SALAD > 101

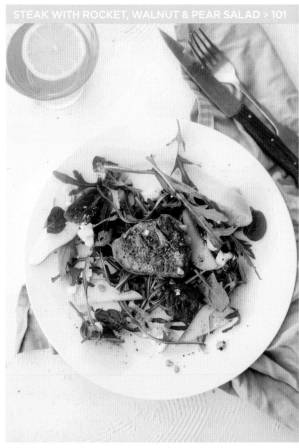

FIVE-WAY STEAK

To me, nothing beats a simple grass-fed steak and LCHF side, especially mid-week when kitchen time is less available. I've included my five favourite options for you to try, but you are really only limited by your imagination here.

STEAK WITH WARM BROCCOLI SALAD

SERVES Ⓕ Ⓜ 2   PREP : 10 MINUTES   COOK : 15 MINUTES

2 tablespoons extra-virgin olive oil / 4 tablespoons extra-virgin olive oil
1 teaspoon sea salt
2 × 120g grass-fed beef eye fillet steaks / 2 × 150g grass-fed beef eye fillet steaks
200g broccoli, cut into florets / 400g broccoli, cut into florets
1 lemon, juiced
1 avocado, diced
2 tablespoons goji berries
60g spinach leaves
¼ cup almonds, roughly chopped
sea salt and pepper, to taste

1 Combine 1 tablespoon oil and salt on a plate and toss steak in marinade.

2 Bring a small saucepan of water to the boil. Place broccoli in a colander or steamer basket, cover with a lid and lightly steam for 4–5 minutes. Remove from the colander or steamer basket and set aside to cool.

3 Combine remaining olive oil and lemon juice in a small bowl and whisk to combine.

4 Place avocado, goji berries, spinach and almonds in a bowl. Toss through

5 broccoli and dressing, and season well with salt and pepper.

6 Heat a barbeque grill or frypan on a medium-high heat and add steak. Cook for 5–7 minutes each side, depending on your desired result. Rest steak for 5 minutes before serving with the salad.

Ⓕ MACROS Cals : **499** CHO : **27g** P : **26g** Fat : **36g**
Ⓜ MACROS Cals : **680** CHO : **34g** P : **33g** Fat : **51g**

STEAK WITH ZUCCHINI & BRUSSELS SPROUTS SALAD

SERVES (F) (M) 2   PREP : 10 MINUTES   COOK : 25 MINUTES

2 zucchinis, cut into 5mm batons
2 cups sliced Brussels sprouts
1 tablespoon cold-pressed extra-
  virgin coconut oil, melted
½ teaspoon chilli flakes
sea salt and pepper, to taste
1 fennel bulb, sliced
60g rocket leaves
½ cup almonds, roughly chopped
½ avocado, diced
60g goat's feta
2 × 120g grass-fed beef eye fillet
  steaks / 2 × 150g grass-fed
  beef eye fillet steaks
Dressing:
1 tablespoon Dijon mustard
1 tablespoon extra-virgin
  olive oil
½ lemon, juiced
¼ teaspoon salt

1 Preheat oven to 180°C and line a baking tray with
   baking paper.

2 In a large bowl, toss zucchini and Brussels sprouts with
   coconut oil and chilli flakes. Season well with salt and
   pepper and bake for 10 minutes, or until tender. Turn
   vegetables, add sliced fennel, and bake for a further
   10 minutes.

3 Place all the dressing ingredients in a bowl and whisk to
   combine.

4 In the large bowl originally used, place rocket, almonds,
   avocado and feta. Once baked, add zucchini, Brussels
   sprouts and fennel. Add dressing and toss to combine.

5 Season steak with salt and add to a barbecue grill or frypan
   on a medium–high heat. Cook for 4 minutes each side, or
   until cooked to your liking. Remove from the heat and rest
   for 5 minutes before serving with the salad.

(F) MACROS Cals : **609** CHO : **26g** P : **40g** Fat : **46g**
(M) MACROS Cals : **835** CHO : **30g** P : **68g** Fat : **54g**

STEAK WITH BEETROOT & ORANGE SALAD

SERVES (F) (M) 2   PREP : 10 MINUTES   COOK : 50 MINUTES

1 bunch baby beetroots,
  trimmed and quartered
3 oranges (2 zested and sliced,
  1 juiced)
2 teaspoons extra-virgin olive
  oil / 2 tablespoons extra-
  virgin olive oil
sea salt and pepper, to taste
60g rocket leaves
60g walnuts, roughly chopped /
  80g walnuts, roughly chopped
60g goat's feta / 80g goat's feta
2 × 120g grass-fed beef eye
  fillet steaks / 2 × 150g grass-
  fed beef eye fillet steaks

1 Preheat oven to 180°C and line a baking tray with
   baking paper.

2 In a large bowl, toss beetroot with the orange zest, juice
   of 1 orange and 1 tablespoon of the olive oil. Season well
   with salt and pepper and spread on the baking tray. Bake
   for 40 minutes or until beetroot is tender.

3 Segment the remaining 2 oranges into slices. Place
   beetroot, orange slices, rocket and walnuts in a large bowl.
   Toss gently with the remaining oil and sprinkle with feta.

4 Season steak with salt and add to a barbecue grill or frypan
   on a medium–high heat. Cook for 4 minutes each side, or
   until cooked to your liking. Remove from the heat, rest for
   5 minutes and serve with the beetroot and orange salad.

(F) MACROS Cals : **575** CHO : **27g** P : **36g** Fat : **39g**
(M) MACROS Cals : **656** CHO : **25g** P : **43g** Fat : **45g**

STEAK WITH PUMPKIN & AVOCADO SALAD

SERVES Ⓕ Ⓜ 2   PREP : 10 MINUTES   COOK : 20 MINUTES

1 tablespoon cold-pressed extra-virgin coconut oil, melted

½ small jap pumpkin, cut into wedges

1 teaspoon chilli flakes

sea salt and pepper, to taste

2 tablespoons extra-virgin olive oil

1 tablespoon apple cider vinegar

60g rocket leaves

1 avocado, diced

1 baby fennel bulb, thinly sliced

2 tablespoons roughly chopped walnuts / ¼ cup roughly chopped walnuts

2 × 120g grass-fed beef eye fillet steaks / 2 × 150g grass-fed beef eye fillet steaks

1 Preheat oven to 180°C and line a baking tray with baking paper.

2 Toss melted coconut oil with pumpkin and chilli flakes and season well with salt and pepper. Transfer to the baking tray and roast for 20 minutes, or until golden.

3 Place olive oil, vinegar and salt to taste in a small bowl, and whisk to combine.

4 In a large bowl, place rocket, avocado, fennel and walnuts. Add roasted pumpkin and dressing and toss gently to combine.

5 Season steak with salt and add to a barbecue grill or frypan on a medium–high heat. Cook for 4 minutes on each side, or until cooked to your liking. Remove from the heat, rest for 5 minutes and serve with the salad.

Ⓕ MACROS Cals : **639** CHO : **13g** P : **28g** Fat : **55g**

Ⓜ MACROS Cals : **755** CHO : **14g** P : **35g** Fat : **64g**

STEAK WITH ROCKET, WALNUT & PEAR SALAD

SERVES Ⓕ Ⓜ 1   PREP : 10 MINUTES + 1–2 HOURS MARINATING   COOK : 10 MINUTES

125g grass-fed beef eye fillet steak / 150g grass-fed beef eye fillet steak

1 tablespoon extra-virgin olive oil / 2 tablespoons extra-virgin olive oil

sea salt and pepper, to taste

ROCKET, WALNUT & PEAR SALAD

150g rocket leaves

1 tablespoon chopped walnuts

30g goat's feta

¼ pear, thinly sliced / ½ pear, thinly sliced

½ lemon, juiced

sea salt and pepper, to taste

1 Marinate steak in olive oil, sea salt and pepper for 1–2 hours.

2 Drain marinade into a preheated frypan over medium–high heat. Add steak and cook for 6–8 minutes per side, or until cooked to your liking. Rest for 5 minutes before serving.

3 Arrange rocket, walnuts, feta and pear in a bowl, and dress with lemon juice, salt and pepper. Serve alongside steak, and enjoy.

Ⓕ MACROS Cals : **565** CHO : **10g** P : **48g** Fat : **32g**

Ⓜ MACROS Cals : **764** CHO : **20g** P : **62g** Fat : **53g**

MEXICAN BEEF TORTILLAS

SERVES (F)♀ (M)♂ 4   PREP : 10 MINUTES   COOK : 8 HOURS

A slow cooker is one of my favourite kitchen tools, as it not only means that dinner is ready when you walk in the door from work, but it's one of the best ways to cook cheaper cuts of meat. This recipe uses chuck steak, but it's just as tender as an eye fillet, especially when cooked on low for eight hours.

1 teaspoon paprika
1 teaspoon chilli powder
1 teaspoon garlic powder
1 teaspoon onion powder
1kg grass-fed chuck steak, whole piece
250g cherry tomatoes, quartered
2 cups beef stock
1 tablespoon coconut aminos
sea salt and pepper, to taste
½ red onion, diced
½ red chilli, deseeded and finely chopped
½ bunch coriander, roughly chopped
1 avocado, diced / 2 avocados, diced
1 lime, juiced
1 tablespoon extra-virgin olive oil / 2 tablespoons extra-virgin olive oil
1 large iceberg lettuce

1 Combine paprika, chilli, garlic powder and onion powder and rub over whole chuck steak. Place in the slow cooker. Add half the cherry tomatoes, plus all the beef stock and aminos. Season well with salt and pepper and turn the slow cooker on to low for 8 hours, or until beef is tender.

2 Leaving the beef in the slow cooker, take two forks and shred the beef.

3 Make a salsa by combining the remaining cherry tomatoes with the red onion, chilli, coriander and avocado. Dress with lime juice and olive oil, and season well with salt and pepper.

4 To serve, select 4 large lettuce leaves. Top with pulled beef and tomato salsa and serve.

(F)♀ MACROS   Cals : **479**   CHO : **11g**   P : **54g**   Fat : **24g**
(M)♂ MACROS   Cals : **568**   CHO : **11g**   P : **54g**   Fat : **24g**

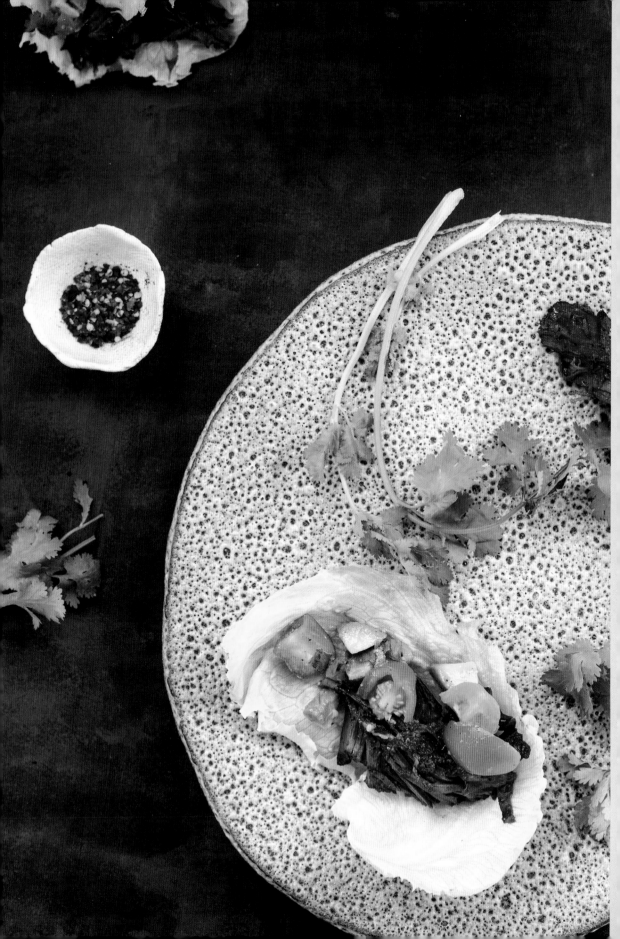

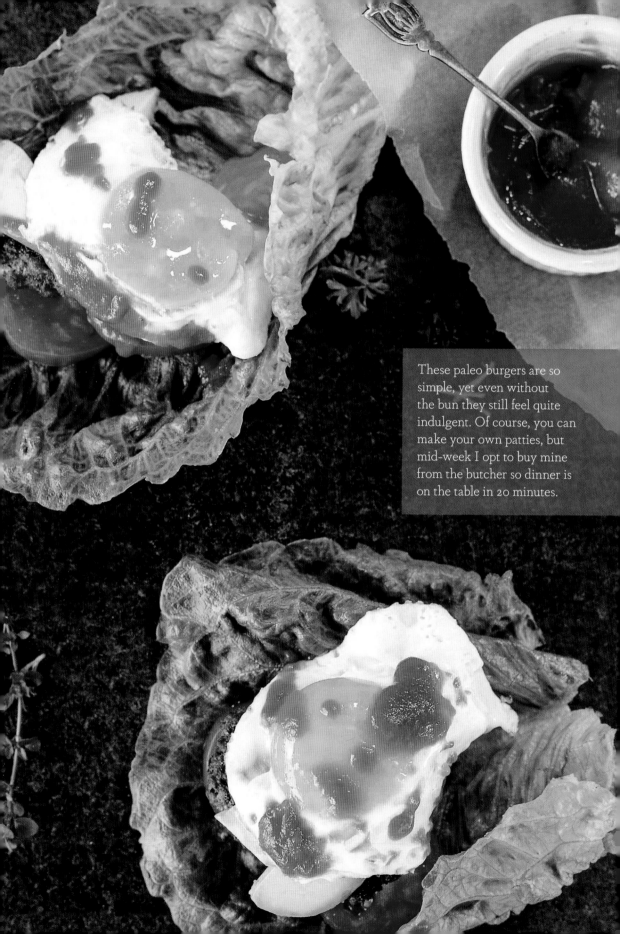

These paleo burgers are so simple, yet even without the bun they still feel quite indulgent. Of course, you can make your own patties, but mid-week I opt to buy mine from the butcher so dinner is on the table in 20 minutes.

PALEO BURGERS #1

SERVES Ⓕ Ⓜ 1   PREP : 10 MINUTES   COOK : 10 MINUTES

1 tablespoon cold-pressed
   extra-virgin coconut oil
1 grass-fed beef patty /
   2 grass-fed beef patties
1 free-range egg / 2 free-range
   eggs
2 large iceberg or cos lettuce
   leaves
½ tomato, sliced
¼ avocado, sliced /
   ½ avocado, sliced
Sugar-free Tomato Sauce
   (see recipe page 205)
sea salt and pepper, to taste

1 Melt oil in a frypan over medium–high heat. Cook beef
   patties and eggs to your liking.

2 Fill lettuce leaves with remaining ingredients and top with
   patties and eggs. If you're happy to get your hands dirty,
   wrap the lettuce leaves around the ingredients to form
   a burger in your hands, and enjoy.

Ⓕ MACROS Cals : **536** CHO : **9g** P : **29g** Fat : **41g**
Ⓜ MACROS Cals : **712** CHO : **9g** P : **48g** Fat : **63g**

PALEO BURGERS #2

SERVES (F)(M) 1   PREP : 10 MINUTES   COOK : 10 MINUTES

1 tablespoon cold-pressed
   extra-virgin coconut oil
1 grass-fed beef patty /
   2 grass-fed beef patties
1 free-range egg
2 small rashers pasture-raised
   bacon
2 large iceberg or cos lettuce
   leaves
½ tomato, sliced
½ avocado, mashed
1 tablespoon kimchi
Sugar-free Tomato Sauce
   (see recipe on page 205)
sea salt and pepper, to taste

1 Melt coconut oil in a frypan over medium–high heat.
   Cook beef patty, egg and bacon to your liking.

2 Fill lettuce leaves with remaining ingredients and top with
   patties, bacon and eggs. If you're happy to get your hands
   dirty, wrap the lettuce leaves around the ingredients to form
   a burger in your hands, and enjoy.

(F) MACROS   Cals : **585**   CHO : **11g**   P : **24g**   Fat : **48g**
(M) MACROS   Cals : **795**   CHO : **11g**   P : **34g**   Fat : **70g**

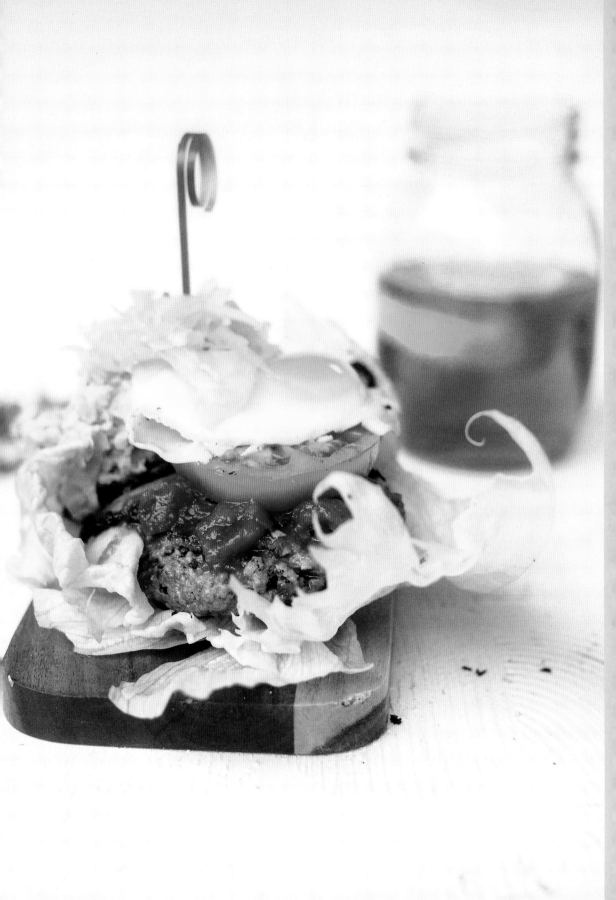

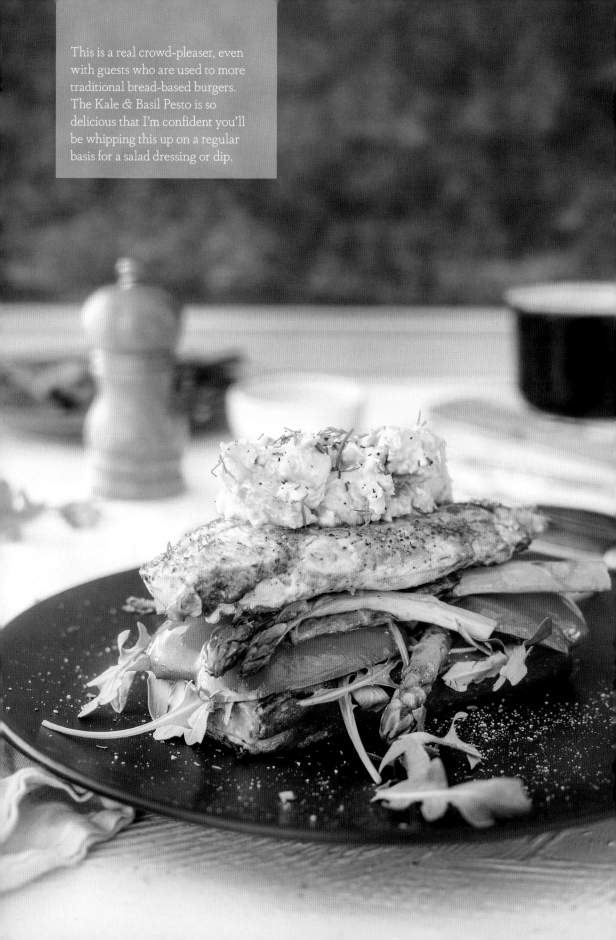

This is a real crowd-pleaser, even with guests who are used to more traditional bread-based burgers. The Kale & Basil Pesto is so delicious that I'm confident you'll be whipping this up on a regular basis for a salad dressing or dip.

PESTO CHICKEN BURGER

SERVES (F)♀ (M)♂ 2   PREP : 40 MINUTES   COOK : 15 MINUTES

4 teaspoons extra-virgin
  olive oil
240g free-range chicken breast
  fillet, cut lengthways /
  300g free-range chicken breast
  fillet, cut lengthways
100g sweet potato
sea salt and pepper, to taste
1 red capsicum, quartered
1 bunch asparagus, cut in half
  lengthways
1 avocado
20g goat's cheese /
  40g goat's cheese
40g rocket leaves
1 tablespoon roughly chopped
  fresh dill

KALE & BASIL PESTO
1 cup chopped kale leaves
  (stalks removed)
1 cup fresh basil leaves
2 tablespoons nutritional yeast
⅔ cup pine nuts
3 tablespoons extra-virgin
  olive oil
1 tablespoon garlic-infused
  extra-virgin olive oil
2 teaspoons lemon juice
sea salt and pepper, to taste

1   To make the Kale & Basil Pesto, place all the ingredients in
    a food processor or blender and blitz to desired consistency.
    Stir in extra lemon juice if required.

2   In a shallow bowl, combine 2 tablespoons of pesto with
    1 teaspoon of olive oil and add the chicken. Toss to combine
    and set aside for 30 minutes to marinate. Store leftover
    pesto in an airtight glass container in the fridge for 5–7 days.

3   Meanwhile, preheat oven to 180°C and line a baking tray
    with baking paper.

4   Slice sweet potato into 3cm-thick slices and place on the
    baking tray. Drizzle with 1 teaspoon of the olive oil and
    season well with salt and pepper. Bake in the oven for
    10 minutes, or until golden.

5   In another bowl, combine remaining oil with capsicum and
    asparagus.

6   Heat a barbeque grill or frypan over medium–high heat
    and cook capsicum and asparagus for 5–8 minutes, or until
    tender and golden. Remove from the heat.

7   Add marinated chicken and cook for 3 minutes each side,
    depending on the thickness of your chicken. Allow to rest
    for 5 minutes.

8   Place avocado and goat's cheese in a small bowl and
    roughly mash together. Season well with salt and pepper.

9   To serve, place sweet potato on the bottom of each plate
    and top with rocket, char-grilled capsicum and asparagus.
    Add chicken and top with mashed avocado and dill, and
    season further if necessary.

(F)♀ MACROS Cals : **569** CHO : **20g** P : **34g** Fat : **29g**
(M)♂ MACROS Cals : **715** CHO : **20g** P : **42g** Fat : **32g**

LCHF SAN CHOY BAU

SERVES (F)(M) 2   PREP : 10 MINUTES   COOK : 15 MINUTES

Traditionally, san choy bau is already a lower-carb menu choice, so I wanted to show you how to improve the quality with this homemade version. You'll notice I use tamari, which is a gluten-free soy replacement, but feel free to use coconut aminos if you prefer to eat soy-free.

1 tablespoon cold-pressed
   extra-virgin coconut oil
250g chicken thigh fillets,
   diced / 300g chicken thigh
   fillets, diced
150g mushrooms, finely diced
20g kale, finely chopped
1 red chilli, deseeded and
   finely chopped
1 tablespoon grated ginger
1 garlic clove, crushed
4 spring onions, thinly sliced
1 tablespoon sesame oil
4 tablespoons tamari
iceberg lettuce leaves
1 tablespoon slivered almonds /
   1½ tablespoons slivered
   almonds
¼ bunch coriander, leaves
   roughly chopped
sea salt, to taste

1 Heat a frypan over medium–high heat and add coconut oil.
2 Add chicken, mushrooms, kale, chilli, ginger, garlic, spring onions, sesame oil and tamari. Sauté for 15 minutes, or until the mushrooms are cooked and the chicken is browned.
3 Separate lettuce leaves for serving. Trim if required, and set aside.
4 To serve, spoon the chicken mixture into the lettuce cups and top with slivered almonds and coriander. Season well with salt.

(F) MACROS Cals : **623** CHO : **19g** P : **43g** Fat : **44g**
(M) MACROS Cals : **795** CHO : **25g** P : **53g** Fat : **57g**

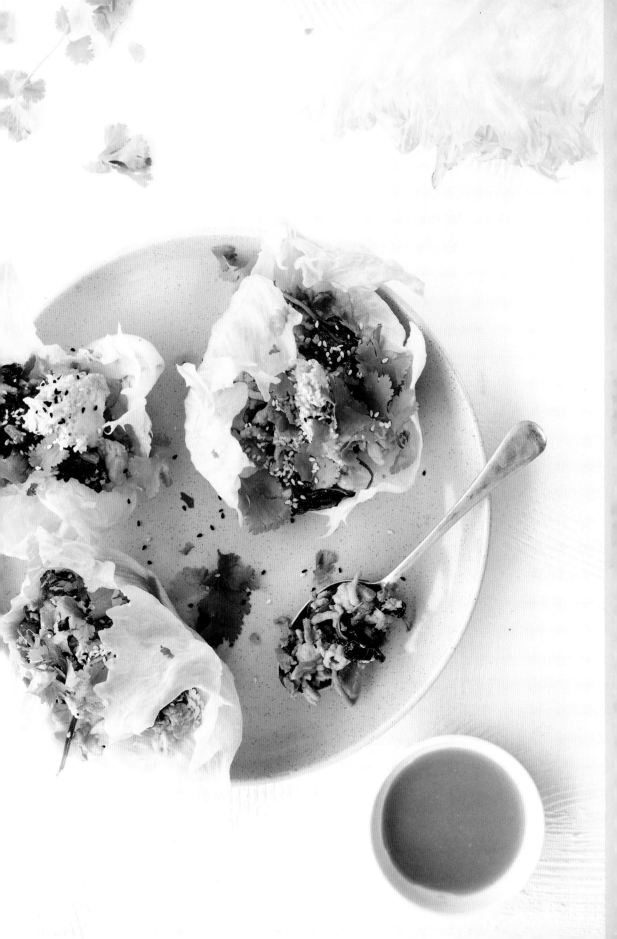

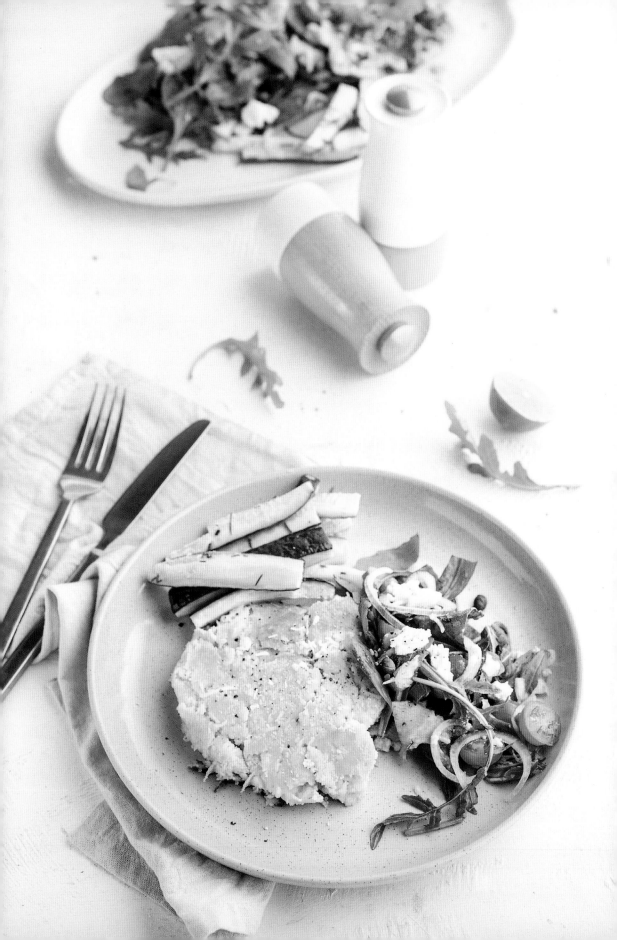

HEALTHY FRIED FISH & ZUCCHINI CHIPS

SERVES Ⓕ Ⓜ 4   PREP : 10 MINUTES   COOK : 20 MINUTES

I'm a huge fan of vegie chips and I love combining these zucchini chips with fresh fish and a side salad. This meal is quick to prepare and never fails to please the whole family.

1 free-range egg
2–3 tablespoons unsweetened
   almond milk
¼ cup coconut flour
½ cup almond meal
2 tablespoons shredded
   coconut
sea salt and pepper, to taste
480g white fish fillets, such
   as flathead / 600g white fish
   fillets, such as flathead
¼ cup cold-pressed extra-virgin
   coconut oil

ZUCCHINI CHIPS
2 large zucchinis, sliced into
   thick, chip-like pieces / 3 large
   zucchinis, sliced into thick,
   chip-like pieces
1 tablespoon cold-pressed
   extra-virgin coconut oil, melted
1 tablespoon roughly chopped
   rosemary
1 teaspoon sea salt

SIDE SALAD
60g rocket and spinach leaves
250g cherry tomatoes, quartered
½ red onion, thinly sliced
4 tablespoons sauerkraut
2 tablespoons capers, drained
25g goat's feta / 50g goat's feta

1. Preheat oven to 160°C and line a baking tray with paper.

2. In a small bowl, whisk the egg together with the almond milk and pour into a shallow dish. Place the coconut flour in another shallow dish. In a third shallow dish add the almond meal and shredded coconut and mix and season well.

3. Place the fish fillets in the coconut flour and gently toss to coat. Dip the fish into the egg mixture and then toss in the almond meal mixture to coat. Repeat this twice and set aside.

4. Toss the zucchini slices with coconut oil, rosemary and salt, place on the baking tray and bake for 10 minutes. Turn the chips, then return to the oven for a further 10 minutes, or until cooked and golden

5. Meanwhile, combine the salad ingredients in a large bowl and divide evenly between serving plates.

6. In a large frypan, melt the oil and cook the fish for 2–3 minutes each side, until golden and cooked through. Serve with the salad and zucchini chips.

Ⓕ MACROS Cals : **584** CHO : **35g** P : **39g** Fat : **40g**
Ⓜ MACROS Cals : **630** CHO : **37g** P : **45g** Fat : **41g**

CLEAN SNAGS WITH PUMPKIN MASH & ASPARAGUS

SERVES Ⓕ Ⓜ 4   PREP : 10 MINUTES   COOK : 15 MINUTES

If you come from a low-fat background, you probably haven't eaten sausages in years (or decades)! These days, provided you buy the right brand, sausages can be of an extremely high quality and made with very few ingredients. They're great to batch-cook – after all, who doesn't love a cold snag straight out of the fridge the next day?

3 bunches asparagus
1 teaspoon extra-virgin olive oil / 1 tablespoon extra-virgin olive oil
½ lemon, juiced
8 grass-fed sausages

PUMPKIN MASH
400g pumpkin, diced
1 tablespoon grass-fed butter / 2 tablespoons grass-fed butter
1 tablespoon unsweetened almond milk
sea salt, to taste
2 cups spinach leaves

1 To make Pumpkin Mash: Bring a small saucepan of water to the boil. Place pumpkin in a colander or steamer basket, cover with a lid and steam for 4–5 minutes. Remove from the colander or steamer basket and return to the drained saucepan. Mash the pumpkin with butter and almond milk and season well with salt. Stir through spinach.

2 Brush asparagus with olive oil and lemon juice.

3 Heat a barbecue grill to medium–hot and char-grill asparagus until tender. Set aside.

4 Add sausages to the grill and cook them slowly, turning every couple of minutes until they are brown all over and cooked through.

5 Serve the sausages alongside the mash and asparagus.

Ⓕ MACROS Cals : **442** CHO : **15g** P : **29g** Fat : **25g**
Ⓜ MACROS Cals : **622** CHO : **15g** P : **29g** Fat : **45g**

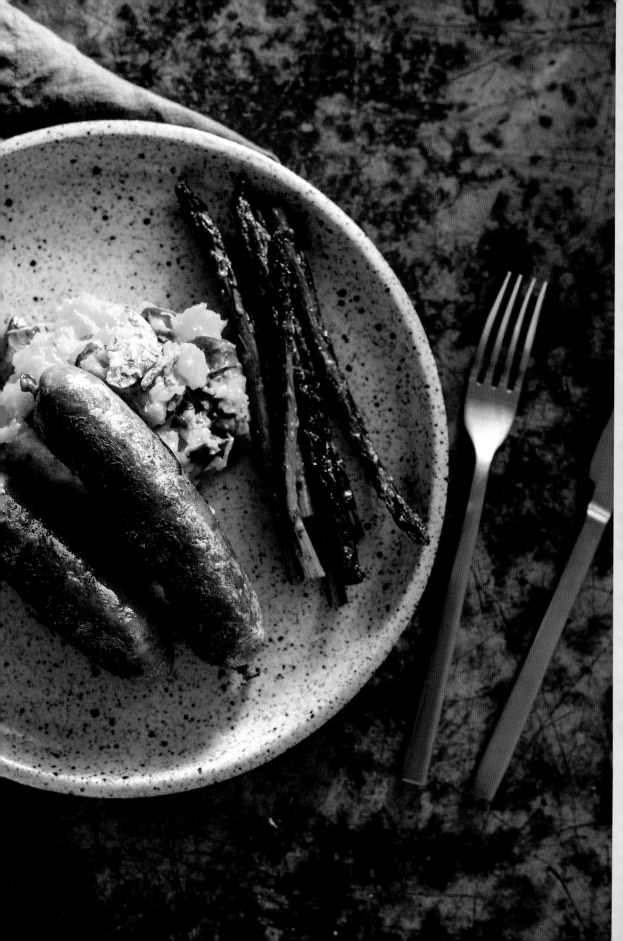

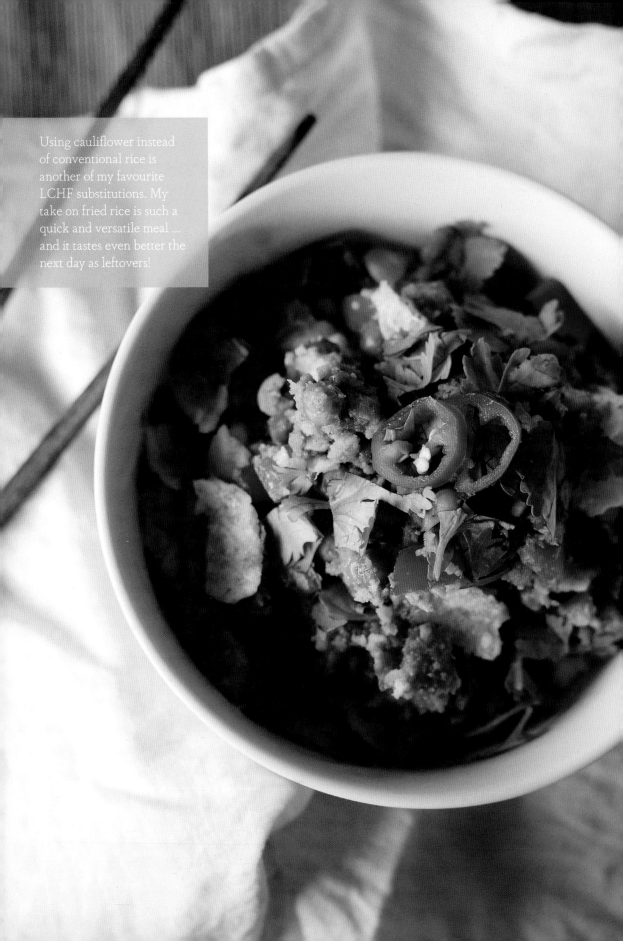

Using cauliflower instead of conventional rice is another of my favourite LCHF substitutions. My take on fried rice is such a quick and versatile meal ... and it tastes even better the next day as leftovers!

CHICKEN 'FRIED RICE'

SERVES Ⓕ Ⓜ 2   PREP : 10 MINUTES   COOK : 15 MINUTES

½ head of broccoli, cut into florets

½ head of cauliflower, cut into florets

2 tablespoons cold-pressed extra-virgin coconut oil / 2½ tablespoons cold-pressed extra-virgin coconut oil

2 free-range eggs, lightly beaten

¼ cup raw cashews

2 rashers pasture-raised bacon, diced

1 red chilli, deseeded and finely chopped

1 red capsicum, diced

1 carrot, diced

2 celery stalks, diced

¼ cup peas

2 tablespoons tamari

1 tablespoon fish sauce

sea salt and pepper, to taste

200g free-range chicken thigh fillets, diced / 300g free-range chicken thigh fillets, diced

1 bunch coriander, roughly chopped

1   Pulse broccoli and cauliflower in a food processor or blender until it resembles rice. Depending on the size of your processor, you may need to split this step into two or three batches to ensure you don't end up with a mash.

2   Heat ½ tablespoon of the coconut oil in a large frypan or wok over medium heat and pour eggs in. Cook as you would an omelette then remove from the pan and dice into small pieces.

3   Add cashews to the pan and lightly toast for 4–5 minutes, or until golden. Remove and set aside.

4   Heat another ½ tablespoon oil and quickly stir-fry bacon and chilli until browned.

5   Add capsicum, carrot, celery and peas, and continue to stir-fry until tender.

6   Add broccoli and cauliflower rice and stir-fry for 2–3 minutes.

7   Stir in tamari and fish sauce and season with well with salt and pepper. Toss through diced egg and serve into two bowls.

8   Heat the frypan or wok over high heat and add remaining coconut oil. Cook chicken for 3 minutes on each side, or until cooked through and golden.

9   Place chicken on top of fried rice and season further if necessary. Top with chopped coriander and the toasted cashews.

Ⓕ MACROS Cals : 656   CHO : 22g   P : 40g   Fat : 46g
Ⓜ MACROS Cals : 706   CHO : 22g   P : 50g   Fat : 47g

VEGETARIAN 'FRIED RICE'

SERVES (F) (M) 2   PREP : 10 MINUTES   COOK : 15 MINUTES

½ medium head of cauliflower,
   cut into florets
2 tablespoons cold-pressed
   extra-virgin coconut oil
1 garlic clove, finely chopped
1 small red chilli, deseeded and
   finely chopped
¼ green capsicum, diced
4 button mushrooms, sliced
½ bunch broccolini, chopped
½ cup fresh peas
2 celery stalks, chopped
2 tablespoons coconut aminos
1 tablespoon fish sauce
sea salt and pepper, to taste
2 free-range eggs, lightly
   beaten

1 Pulse cauliflower in a food processor or blender until it
   resembles rice. Depending on the size of your processor,
   you may need to split this step into two or three batches
   to ensure you don't end up with a mash.

2 Heat 1 tablespoon of the coconut oil in a frypan over
   medium–high heat and lightly brown garlic.

3 Add chilli, capsicum, mushrooms, broccolini, peas and
   celery and stir well.

4 Add coconut aminos, fish sauce and salt and pepper, and
   toss to combine.

5 Add cauliflower rice and sauté for 2–3 minutes, keeping
   vegetables crunchy.

6 Serve into two bowls.

7 In a frypan, heat remaining coconut oil over medium heat
   and pour eggs in. Cook as you would an omelette then
   remove from the pan, dice into small pieces and stir
   through the bowls of fried rice. Enjoy.

(F) MACROS Cals : **561** CHO : **24g** P : **15g** Fat : **44g**

(M) MACROS Cals : **561** CHO : **24g** P : **15g** Fat : **44g**

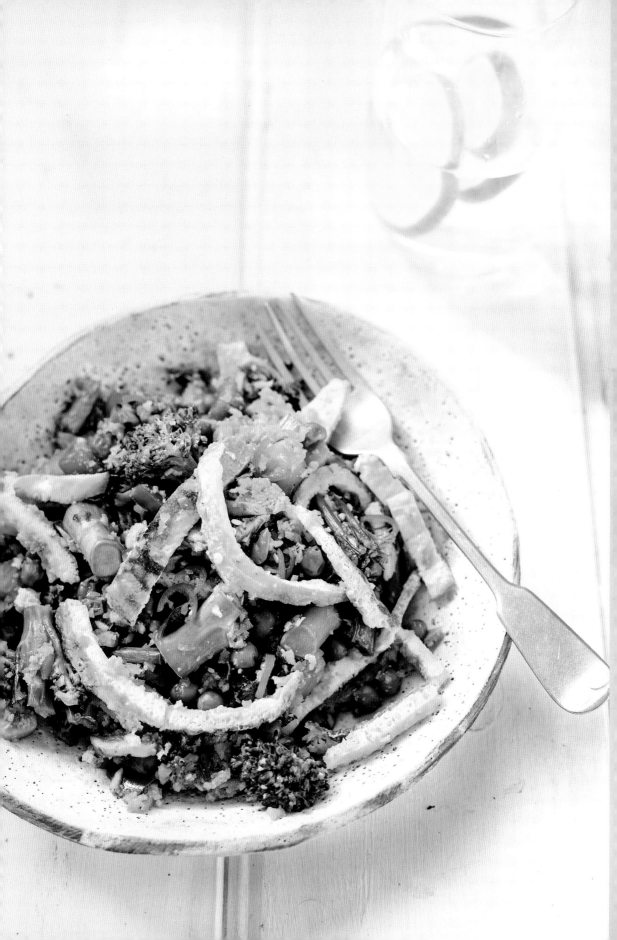

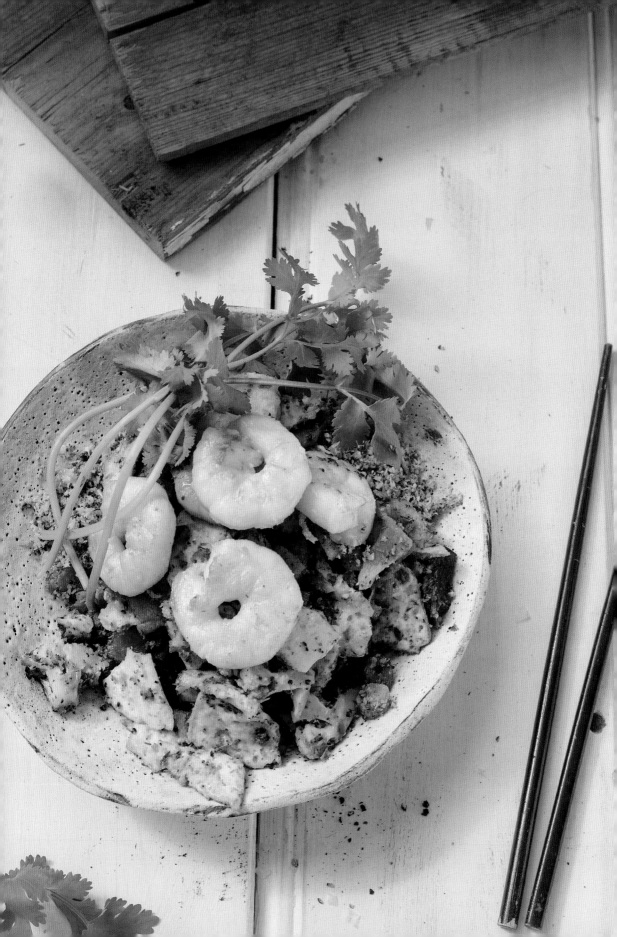

LOW CARB SEAFOOD 'FRIED RICE'

SERVES (F) (M) 4 / 2   PREP : 10 MINUTES   COOK : 15 MINUTES

1 head of broccoli, cut into florets
2 tablespoons cold-pressed extra-virgin coconut oil
4 free-range eggs, lightly beaten
3 rashers pasture-raised bacon, diced
1 red chilli, deseeded and finely diced
1 red capsicum, diced
1 carrot, diced
1 cup roughly chopped cauliflower
3 celery stalks, diced
½ cup peas
300g fresh green prawns, peeled and deveined
2 tablespoons tamari
1 tablespoon fish sauce
sea salt and pepper, to taste
1 bunch coriander, roughly chopped

1   Pulse broccoli in a food processor or blender until it resembles rice. Depending on the size of your processor, you may need to split this step into two or three batches to ensure you don't end up with a mash.

2   Heat 1 tablespoon of the coconut oil in a large frypan or wok over medium–high heat and pour eggs in. Cook as you would an omelette then remove from the pan and dice into small pieces.

3   Heat the remaining oil and quickly stir-fry bacon and chilli until browned.

4   Add capsicum, carrot, cauliflower, celery and peas, and continue to stir-fry until tender.

5   Add prawns and stir-fry for 5–6 minutes, or until cooked through.

6   Add broccoli rice, tamari and fish sauce, and season well with salt and pepper. Toss well for 2–3 minutes to ensure ingredients are well combined.

7   Turn the mixture into bowls, toss through the diced egg and serve topped with coriander.

(F) MACROS   Cals : 293   CHO : 13g   P : 28g   Fat : 14g
(M) MACROS   Cals : 587   CHO : 26g   P : 56g   Fat : 27g

GREEN CHICKEN CURRY
WITH CAULIFLOWER RICE

SERVES (F) (M) 4   PREP : 10 MINUTES   COOK : 30 MINUTES

This is a much-loved staple in my household because it's easy to batch-cook, reheats extremely well and tastes amazing. I find it so rewarding to make curry paste from scratch rather than relying on ready-made products, which are usually packed with sugar and vegetable oil.

2 green chillies, deseeded
  and finely chopped
2 cloves garlic
1 stalk lemongrass, sliced
1 tablespoon curry powder
1 tablespoon turmeric
¼ cup cold-pressed extra-virgin
  coconut oil, plus 1 tablespoon
  extra, for cooking
400ml coconut milk
400ml coconut cream
1 small sweet potato, peeled
  and roughly chopped
500g free-range chicken thigh
  fillets, diced
1 bunch broccolini
1 zucchini, diced
sea salt and pepper, to taste
1 head of cauliflower, cut
  into florets
¼ bunch coriander, leaves
  roughly chopped
1 lemon, cut into wedges

1 In a blender, place chilli, garlic, lemongrass, curry powder, turmeric and the ¼ cup coconut oil. Blitz until a paste forms. If you are unfamiliar with lemongrass, simply remove the tough outer leaves and the bulb (end), and slice the stalk using all of the fleshy pale part. Stop slicing when you get to the greener, more woody section.

2 Heat the remaining 1 tablespoon oil in a large frypan over medium–high heat and stir-fry the curry paste for 2 minutes, or until it becomes fragrant.

3 Stir in coconut milk, coconut cream, sweet potato and chicken. Simmer for 15 minutes, or until chicken is cooked and sweet potato is soft.

4 Stir in broccolini and zucchini and simmer for 5 minutes. Season well with salt and pepper.

5 To make cauliflower rice: Pulse cauliflower in a food processor or blender until it resembles rice. Depending on the size of your processor, you may need to split this step into two or three batches to ensure you don't end up with a mash. Heat remaining oil in a large frypan over medium heat and lightly sauté cauliflower rice for 2–3 minutes, or until soft.

6 Serve curry on top of cauliflower rice with fresh coriander and a lemon wedge. Leftovers will keep in the fridge for 3–4 days.

(F) MACROS Cals : **676** CHO : **29g** P : **40g** Fat : **38g**
(M) MACROS Cals : **676** CHO : **29g** P : **40g** Fat : **38g**

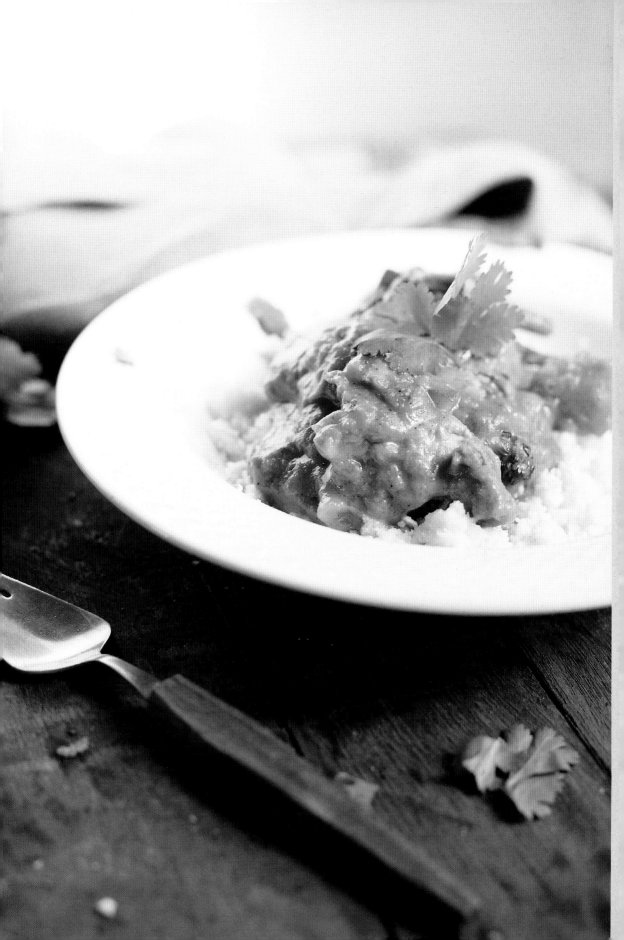

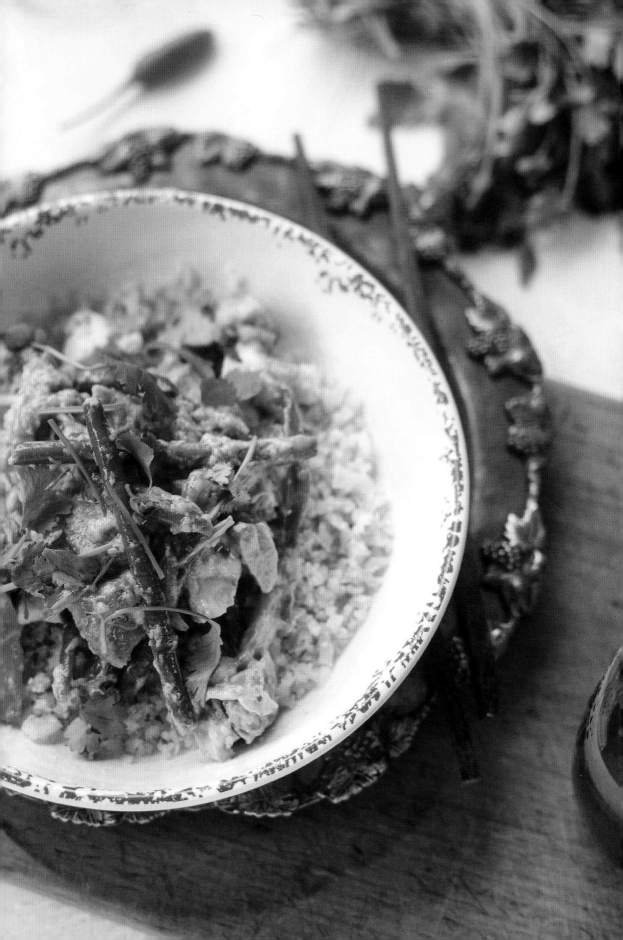

CHICKEN SATAY STIR-FRY WITH CAULIFLOWER RICE

SERVES Ⓕ Ⓜ 4   PREP : 10 MINUTES   COOK : 10 MINUTES

A healthy satay?! Yes please! It's almost hard to believe that this could be good for you, but I assure you it is. For variety, I've chosen to use almond butter to make the satay sauce, but peanut butter also works really well.

1 tablespoon cold-pressed extra-virgin coconut oil / 2 tablespoons cold-pressed extra-virgin coconut oil
500g free-range chicken thigh fillets, diced / 600g free-range chicken thigh fillets, diced
1 red capsicum, cut into strips
1 carrot, cut into strips
1 cup broccoli florets
½ cup green beans
¼ cup chicken broth
sea salt and pepper, to taste
1 head of cauliflower, cut into florets
¼ bunch coriander, roughly chopped

SATAY SAUCE
¼ cup almond butter
1 teaspoon coconut aminos
½ teaspoon garlic powder, or 1 garlic clove
1 tablespoon grated ginger
3 tablespoons coconut cream
½ teaspoon chilli flakes
1 lime, juiced
1 teaspoon raw honey, optional
sea salt, to taste

1. To make the satay sauce, combine all the sauce ingredients in a food processor or blender and blend until smooth. Set aside.

2. Heat half the coconut oil in a wok over medium–high heat and add chicken, stir-frying quickly for 5 minutes, or until browned and cooked through. Remove from the wok and set aside.

3. Add capsicum, carrot, broccoli and beans to the wok and stir-fry for 1 minute.

4. Stir in chicken broth and simmer until vegetables are tender.

5. Add cooked chicken and toss through 3–4 tablespoons of the satay sauce. Season well with salt and pepper.

6. To make cauliflower rice: Pulse cauliflower in a food processor or blender until it resembles rice. Depending on the size of your processor, you may need to split this step into two or three batches to ensure you don't end up with a mash. Heat remaining oil in a large frypan over medium heat and lightly sauté cauliflower rice for 2–3 minutes, or until soft.

7. To serve, place chicken and vegetables on top of a serve of cauliflower rice and top with chopped coriander. Remaining satay sauce can be kept in the fridge for up to 5 days.

Ⓕ MACROS Cals : **441** CHO : **32g** P : **36g** Fat : **24g**
Ⓜ MACROS Cals : **500** CHO : **32g** P : **41g** Fat : **29g**

SUPER-EASY CHICKEN STIR-FRY WITH CAULIFLOWER RICE

SERVES ⓕ ⓜ 2   PREP : 10 MINUTES   COOK : 10 MINUTES

1 head of cauliflower, cut into
    florets
2 tablespoons cold-pressed
    extra-virgin coconut oil
sea salt and pepper, to taste
1 teaspoon extra-virgin olive
    oil / 1 tablespoon extra-virgin
    olive oil
1 brown onion, finely diced
2 garlic cloves, crushed
1 teaspoon grated ginger
250g free-range chicken breast
    fillets, diced / 300g free-range
    chicken breast fillets, diced
1 red capsicum, sliced
1 zucchini, thinly siced
2 bunches bok choy, quartered

SAUCE
1 tablespoon tapioca flour
¼ cup chicken stock
1 garlic clove, crushed
1 tablespoon tamari
1 tablespoon extra-virgin
    olive oil
1 chilli, deseeded and finely
    chopped

TO SERVE
2 tablespoons black sesame
    seeds
½ cup roughly chopped
    coriander

1   In a small bowl, place all the sauce ingredients and mix
    until well combined.

2   To make cauliflower rice: Pulse cauliflower in a food
    processor or blender until it resembles rice. Depending
    on the size of your processor, you may need to split this
    step into two or three batches to ensure you don't end
    up with a mash.

3   Place a large frypan over medium–high heat, add coconut
    oil and cauliflower rice and sauté for 2–3 minutes. Season
    well with salt and pepper and set aside.

4   Add olive oil to the frypan and sauté onion, garlic
    and ginger for 2–3 minutes. Add chicken and stir-fry for
    3 minutes, or until the chicken is golden brown.

5   Add capsicum, zucchini, bok choy and sauce, and stir-fry
    for another 3–4 minutes, or until vegetables are tender.
    Season well with salt and pepper.

6   Serve the stir-fry on top of cauliflower rice and top with
    sesame seeds and chopped coriander.

ⓕ MACROS Cals : **625** CHO : **41g** P : **41g** Fat : **34g**
ⓜ MACROS Cals : **633** CHO : **41g** P : **46g** Fat : **44g**

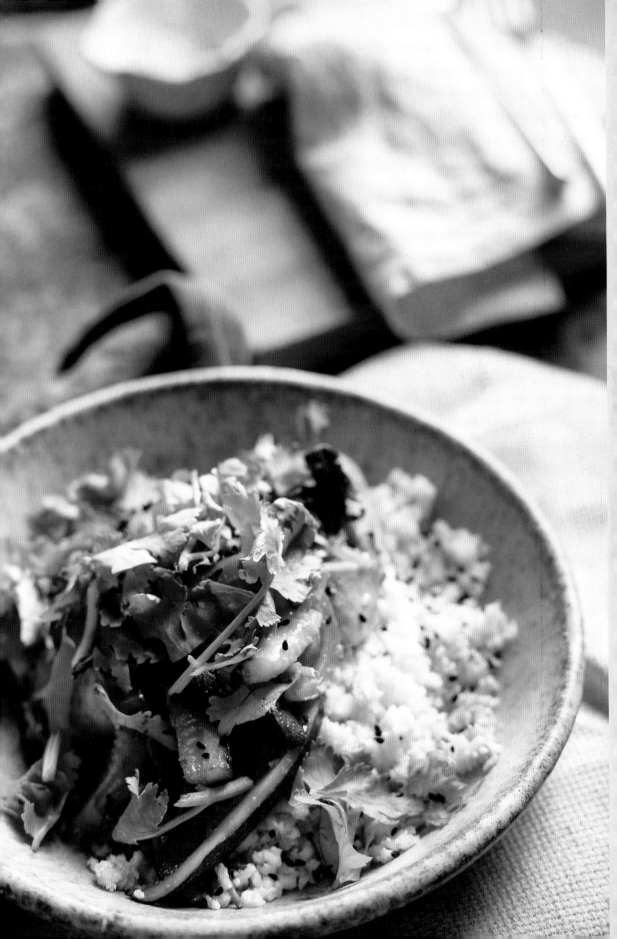

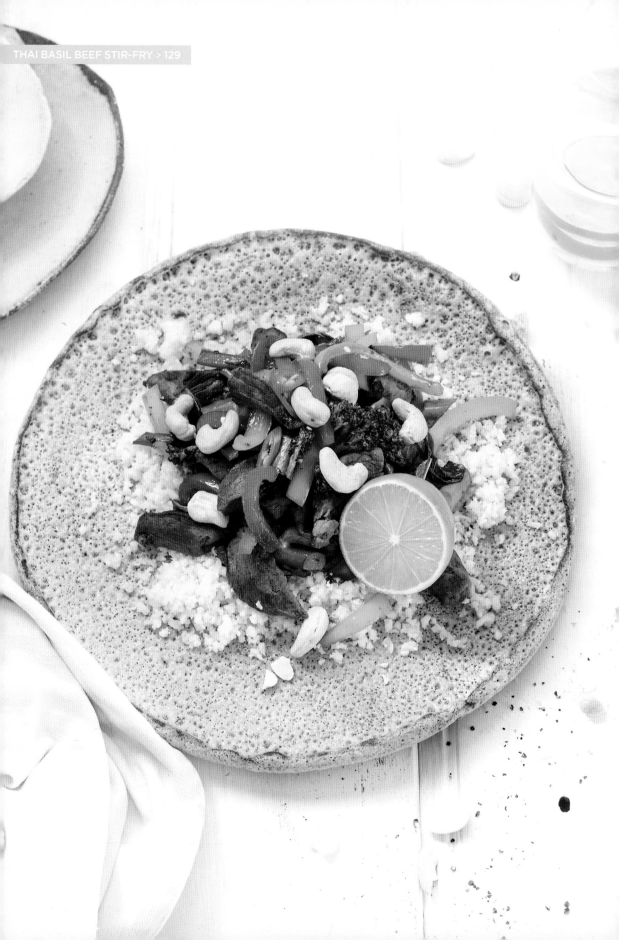

THAI BASIL BEEF STIR-FRY

SERVES (F) (M) 2   PREP : 10 MINUTES   COOK : 10 MINUTES

1 head of cauliflower, cut
  into florets
1 tablespoon cold-pressed
  extra-virgin coconut oil
sea salt and pepper, to taste
2 tablespoons extra-virgin
  olive oil
240g grass-fed beef strips /
  300g grass-fed beef strips
1 red capsicum, sliced
1 yellow capsicum, sliced
1 bunch broccolini, chopped
1 tablespoon fish sauce
12 Thai basil leaves

TO SERVE
1 lime, juiced
1 small red chilli, deseeded
  and sliced
30g raw cashews

1   To make cauliflower rice: Pulse cauliflower in a food
    processor or blender until it resembles rice. Depending on
    the size of your processor, you may need to split this step into
    two or three batches to ensure you don't end up with a mash.

2   Place a wok over medium–high heat, add coconut oil and
    cauliflower rice and sauté for 2–3 minutes. Season well with
    salt and pepper and set aside.

3   Reheat the wok over high heat. Add olive oil and beef strips,
    stir-frying for 5 minutes, or until browned. Remove from
    wok and set aside in a warm place.

4   Add capsicums and broccolini to wok and stir-fry for a few
    minutes until beginning to soften. Return beef to wok with
    fish sauce and basil leaves and stir-fry for another minute.

5   Serve on top of the cauliflower rice with lime juice, chilli
    and cashews.

(F) MACROS   Cals : **773**   CHO : **31g**   P : **77g**   Fat : **47g**
(M) MACROS   Cals : **875**   CHO : **43g**   P : **65g**   Fat : **60g**

CHICKEN & CASHEW STIR-FRY

SERVES (F) (M) 2   PREP : 10 MINUTES   COOK : 10 MINUTES

⅓ cup raw cashews / ½ cup
  raw cashews
1 tablespoon cold-pressed
  extra-virgin coconut oil
1 red onion, cut into wedges
1 garlic clove, crushed
1 red chilli, deseeded and
  finely chopped
300g free-range chicken thigh
  fillets, diced
1 bunch broccolini, roughly
  chopped
1 carrot, sliced
1 red capsicum, sliced
1 yellow capsicum, sliced
1 tablespoon tamari
sea salt and pepper, to taste
¼ bunch coriander, roughly
  chopped

1   Heat a wok or frypan over medium heat and add cashews.
    Toast for 2 minutes, or until lightly golden. Set aside.

2   Heat coconut oil in the pan, add onion, garlic and chilli, and
    sauté for 2–3 minutes or until starting to soften.

3   Add chicken and stir-fry for 5–6 minutes or until golden and
    cooked through.

4   Add remaining vegetables and sauté for 5 minutes, or until
    the vegetables have started to soften yet remain crunchy.

5   Stir through the tamari and cashews and season well with
    salt and pepper.

6   Sprinkle coriander on top of the stir-fry and serve.

(F) MACROS   Cals : **484**   CHO : **24g**   P : **41g**   Fat : **26g**
(M) MACROS   Cals : **538**   CHO : **26g**   P : **43g**   Fat : **30g**

SALMON ON PEA MASH

SERVES (F) (M) 2   PREP : 5 MINUTES   COOK : 15 MINUTES

Another meal that will be on your table in 20 minutes. I often find myself whipping this one up when my vegetable drawer is a little the worse for wear. Keeping frozen salmon and a bag of frozen peas as staples will mean that you're never tempted by greasy takeaway on a Thursday or Friday evening.

200g frozen peas
30g grass-fed butter
1 teaspoon chopped fresh parsley
1 lemon, zested and juiced
1 tablespoon cold-pressed extra-virgin coconut oil
2 × 120g salmon fillets, preferably wild caught / 2 × 150g salmon fillets, preferably wild caught
sea salt and pepper, to taste
1 teaspoon extra-virgin olive oil

1 Bring a small saucepan of water to the boil. Place peas in a colander or steamer basket, cover with a lid and steam for 4–5 minutes. Remove from the colander or steamer basket and return to the drained saucepan.

2 Add butter to the peas and stir to combine. Add parsley, lemon zest and juice and roughly mash with a fork.

3 Heat coconut oil in a medium frypan over medium–high heat and add salmon fillets, skin side down. Season with salt and cook for 5 minutes, or until skin is crispy, then flip the salmon and continue cooking the other side to your liking.

4 Divide pea mash evenly between two plates and place a salmon fillet on top. Season well with salt and pepper and drizzle olive oil on top.

(F) MACROS Cals : 521   CHO : 15g   P : 34g   Fat : 35g
(M) MACROS Cals : 641   CHO : 15g   P : 48g   Fat : 42g

WARM CHICKEN SALAD

SERVES (F) (M) 2   PREP : 10 MINUTES   COOK : 10 MINUTES

250g free-range chicken breast fillet, diced / 300g free-range chicken breast fillet, diced
1 tablespoon Moroccan seasoning
1 tablespoon cold-pressed extra-virgin coconut oil
2 rashers pasture-raised bacon, diced / 4 rashers pasture-raised bacon, diced
1 avocado, diced
125g cherry tomatoes, quartered
1 red capsicum, diced
60g spinach and rocket leaves
1 tablespoon avocado oil
1 tablespoon sunflower seeds
1 tablespoon sesame seeds

1 Place chicken and Moroccan seasoning in a bowl and toss well to combine.

2 Heat a frypan over medium heat and melt coconut oil. Add chicken and sauté for 4–5 minutes, or until golden and cooked through. Set aside.

3 Add bacon to the pan and fry until golden.

4 In a large bowl, place avocado, cherry tomatoes, capsicum and the spinach and rocket leaves. Toss through chicken and bacon and season well with salt and pepper. Drizzle with avocado oil and top with sunflower and sesame seeds.

(F) MACROS Cals : 585   CHO : 15g   P : 36g   Fat : 42g
(M) MACROS Cals : 691   CHO : 15g   P : 45g   Fat : 49g

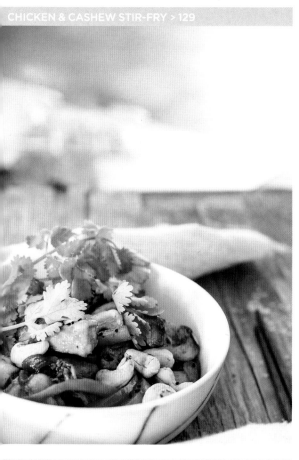

CHICKEN & CASHEW STIR-FRY > 129

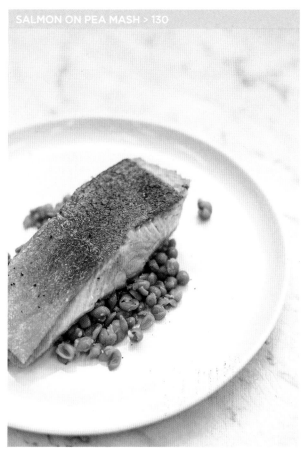

SALMON ON PEA MASH > 130

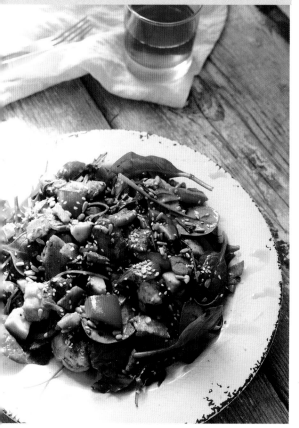

WARM CHICKEN SALAD > 130

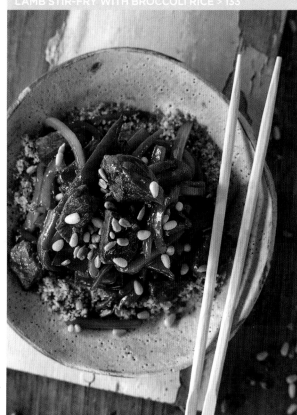

LAMB STIR-FRY WITH BROCCOLI RICE > 133

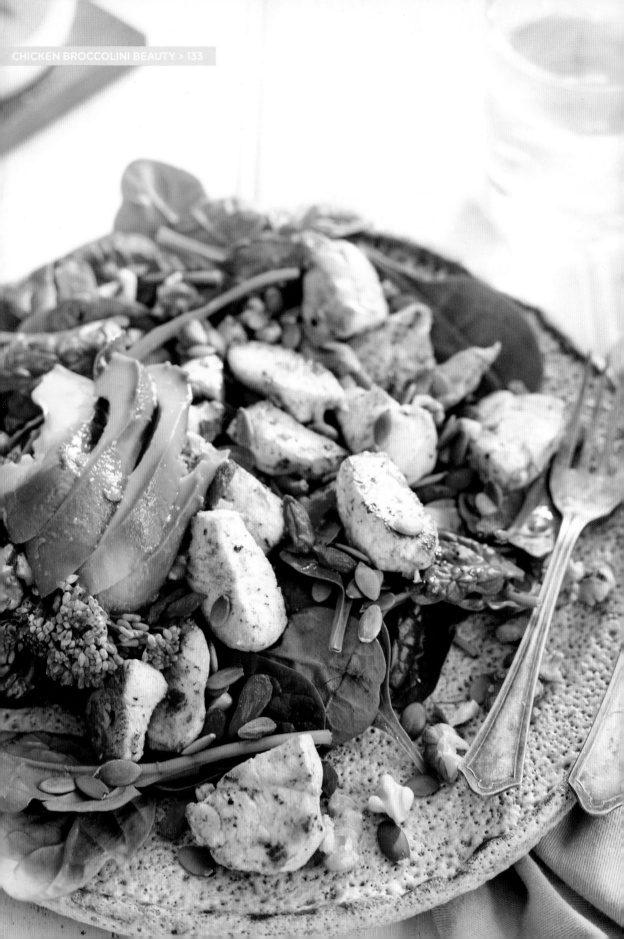

LAMB STIR-FRY WITH BROCCOLI RICE

SERVES (F) (M) 2   PREP : 10 MINUTES   COOK : 10 MINUTES

2 tablespoons tamari
2 teaspoons tapioca flour
¼ teaspoon bicarbonate of soda
1 small head of broccoli, cut
   into florets
2 tablespoons cold-pressed
   extra-virgin coconut oil /
   3 tablespoons cold-pressed
   extra-virgin coconut oil
1 red chilli, deseeded and
   finely chopped
300g lamb backstrap, diced
1 celery stalk, sliced
1 carrot, sliced
1 red capsicum, sliced
1 yellow capsicum, sliced
80g snow peas, trimmed
   and halved lengthways
40g pine nuts / ¼ cup pine nuts
sea salt and pepper, to taste

1 In a small bowl, combine tamari, tapioca flour and
   bicarbonate of soda and set aside.

2 To make the broccoli rice: Pulse broccoli in a food processor
   or blender until it resembles rice. Depending on the size
   of your processor, you may need to split this step into two
   or three batches to ensure you don't end up with a mash.
   Heat 1 tablespoon of the coconut oil in a large frypan over
   medium heat, lightly sauté broccoli rice for 2–3 minutes
   and set aside.

3 Heat a wok over medium heat, add the remaining coconut
   oil plus the chilli, and stir-fry for 1 minute. Add diced lamb
   and stir-fry for 4 minutes, or until browned.

4 Add remaining vegetables and continue to stir-fry for a
   further 5 minutes, or until they are cooked to your liking.

5 Toss through tamari mixture and stir-fry for a further
   1 minute to ensure all ingredients are combined.

6 Serve lamb stir-fry on top of broccoli rice, top with pine
   nuts and season well.

(F) MACROS Cals : **511** CHO : **24g** P : **41g** Fat : **36g**
(M) MACROS Cals : **623** CHO : **27g** P : **45g** Fat : **49g**

CHICKEN BROCCOLINI BEAUTY

SERVES (F) (M) 1   PREP : 10 MINUTES   COOK : 10 MINUTES

1 bunch broccolini
1 teaspoon cold-pressed
   extra-virgin coconut oil
120g free-range chicken thigh
   fillets, diced / 150g free-range
   chicken thigh fillets, diced
150g mixed leafy greens
½ avocado, sliced
sea salt and pepper, to taste
1 tablespoon chopped walnuts
1 teaspoon pumpkin seeds
1 teaspoon goji berries
1 tablespoon apple cider
   vinegar
1 tablespoon extra-virgin
   olive oil

1 Bring a small saucepan of water to the boil. Place broccolini
   in a colander or steamer basket, cover with a lid and steam
   for 4–5 minutes. Remove from the colander or steamer
   basket and set aside to cool.

2 Heat the coconut oil in a frypan over medium heat and fry
   chicken for 3–4 minutes, or until cooked through. Set aside
   to cool.

3 In a large bowl, arrange leafy greens. Add avocado and
   chicken and carefully fold through.

4 Place broccolini on top. Season well and sprinkle with
   walnuts, pumpkin seeds and goji berries. Combine vinegar
   and oil and drizzle over the salad.

(F) MACROS Cals : **518** CHO : **19g** P : **39g** Fat : **43g**
(M) MACROS Cals : **601** CHO : **20g** P : **48g** Fat : **41g**

BAKED FISH WITH TAHINI

SERVES Ⓕ Ⓜ 2   PREP : 10 MINUTES   COOK : 10 MINUTES

Have I mentioned how much I love tahini? My Tahini Dressing (see below) pairs surprisingly well with white fish and, when served with a simple side salad, this is a slightly more creative but still perfect mid-week meal.

240g boneless fish such as
   barramundi / 300g boneless
   fish such as barramundi
sea salt and pepper, to taste

TAHINI DRESSING
1 tablespoon tahini
2 tablespoons extra-virgin
   olive oil
2 tablespoons apple cider
   vinegar
1 lemon, juiced
sea salt and pepper, to taste

TO SERVE
40g rocket leaves
6 cherry tomatoes, quartered
30g chopped walnuts
½ avocado, diced

1 Preheat oven to 200°C.

2 Take two pieces of foil, large enough to wrap each fish fillet, and line each with a square of baking paper.

3 Place the fish, skin side down, on the baking paper. Season well with salt and pepper.

4 Wrap the fish in foil to form a parcel, sealing the edges by folding over the foil, and place on a baking tray. Bake for about 10 minutes. Check the fish and, if not cooked to your liking, simple re-seal the foil and place back in the oven for a few extra minutes.

5 To make the Tahini Dressing, place all the dressing ingredients plus 1 tablespoon water in a small bowl and whisk to combine. If you would like the consistency to be thinner, whisk in a little extra water.

6 To serve, toss together rocket, cherry tomatoes, walnuts and avocado and divide between two plates. Place the fish on top of the salad and drizzle with Tahini Dressing to taste. Store any remaining dressing in an airtight glass jar in the fridge for 5 days.

Ⓕ MACROS Cals : **608** CHO : **13g** P : **42g** Fat : **45g**
Ⓜ MACROS Cals : **632** CHO : **13g** P : **48g** Fat : **45g**

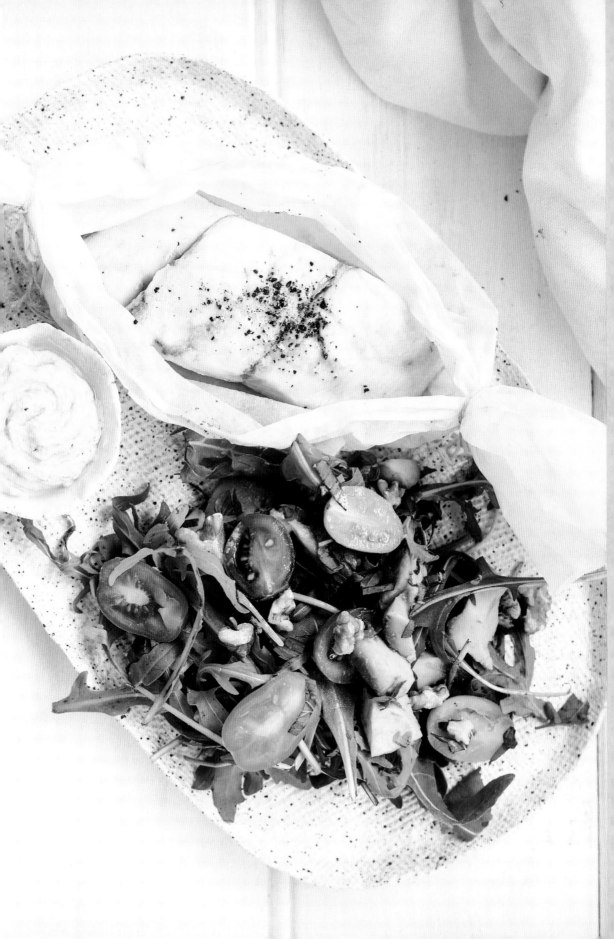

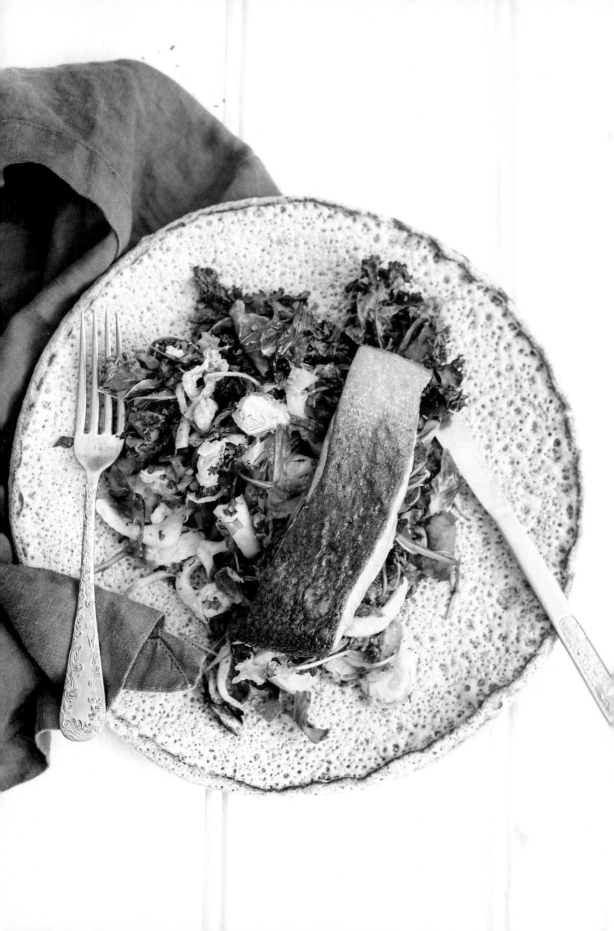

SALMON FILLET WITH ROASTED BRUSSELS SPROUTS & FENNEL SALAD

SERVES Ⓕ Ⓜ 2   PREP : 10 MINUTES   COOK : 20 MINUTES

Brussels sprouts are one of the more polarising vegetables; if you don't like them it's usually because you were forced to eat them overcooked and soggy as a child. When Brussels sprouts are cooked the right way, you'll be pleased to see them back on your plate. Even if you're the biggest Brussels sprout skeptic, I encourage you to try this recipe at least once.

2 tablespoons cold-pressed extra-virgin coconut oil / 4 tablespoons cold-pressed extra-virgin coconut oil

16 Brussels sprouts

1 fennel bulb, thinly sliced

1 teaspoon sea salt, plus extra for seasoning

½ teaspoon chilli flakes

½ bunch kale, stalks removed, leaves roughly chopped

2 × 120g salmon fillets, preferably wild caught / 2 × 150g salmon fillets, preferably wild caught

40g rocket leaves

2 tablespoons walnuts, roughly chopped / ¼ cup walnuts, roughly chopped

extra-virgin olive oil, to taste

sea salt and pepper, to taste

1 Preheat oven to 180°C and line a baking tray with baking paper.

2 In a large bowl, place 1 tablespoon coconut oil, Brussels sprouts, fennel, salt and chilli flakes. Toss to combine and transfer to the baking tray, in a single layer.

3 Roast for 10 minutes, add kale leaves, toss well and return to the oven for 10 minutes.

4 Heat remaining oil in a medium frypan over medium–high heat and add salmon fillets, skin side down. Season with salt and cook for 5 minutes, or until skin is crispy, then flip the salmon and continue cooking the other side to your liking.

5 Place the roasted vegetables in a large bowl. Toss through rocket leaves and walnuts, drizzle with olive oil and season well with salt and pepper. Serve salmon on top.

Ⓕ MACROS Cals : 608 CHO : 27g P : 38g Fat : 41g
Ⓜ MACROS Cals : 788 CHO : 28g P : 39g Fat : 60g

CRISPY SALMON SALAD

SERVES Ⓕ Ⓜ 2   PREP : 10 MINUTES   COOK : 10 MINUTES

1 bunch asparagus, halved
1 avocado
1 tablespoon roughly chopped
   fresh dill
1 lemon, juiced
sea salt and pepper, to taste
1 tablespoon cold-pressed
   extra-virgin olive oil
2 × 120g salmon fillets,
   preferably wild caught /
   2 × 150g salmon fillets,
   preferably wild caught
1 red chilli, deseeded and
   finely chopped
½ bunch kale, stalks removed,
   leaves roughly chopped

1 Bring a small saucepan of water to the boil. Place asparagus
   in a colander or steamer basket, cover with a lid and steam
   for 2–3 minutes. Remove from the colander or steamer
   basket and set aside.

2 In a bowl, roughly mash avocado together with dill and half
   the juiced lemon. Season well with salt and pepper and set
   aside.

3 Heat olive oil in a large frypan over medium–high heat
   and add salmon fillets, skin side down. Season with salt
   and cook for 5 minutes, or until skin is crispy, then flip the
   salmon and continue cooking the other side to your liking.

4 Return salmon to skin side down and flake the flesh with
   a fork, cooking for a further minute in the natural oil of the
   salmon. Add chilli, asparagus and kale, toss to combine,
   and season well with salt and pepper. Cook for a further
   2 minutes.

5 Serve topped with mashed avocado and and the remaining
   lemon juice, if desired.

Ⓕ MACROS Cals : **460** CHO : **12g**   P : **28g** Fat : **33g**
Ⓜ MACROS Cals : **522** CHO : **12g**   P : **34g** Fat : **37g**

ONE-PAN BUTTERFLIED CHICKEN WITH VEGIES

SERVES Ⓕ♀ Ⓜ♂ 6 / 4   PREP : 10 MINUTES   COOK : 50 MINUTES

1 lemon, juiced
2 tablespoons roughly chopped fresh parsley
2 tablespoons fresh thyme leaves
3 tablespoons extra-virgin olive oil
1 whole free-range chicken, approximately 1.8kg, butterflied by your butcher
sea salt and pepper, to taste
2 red onions, cut into wedges
4 carrots, cut into 5cm chunks
½ jap pumpkin, cut into wedges
3 zucchinis, cut into 4cm chunks
60g rocket leaves
2 avocados, diced /
   1 avocado, diced

1 Preheat oven to 180°C and line a roasting tray with baking paper.

2 In a bowl, combine lemon juice, parsley, thyme and 2 tablespoons of the olive oil.

3 Place the chicken flat on the roasting tray. Score the drumsticks with a paring knife and rub the lemon mixture over the entire chicken. Season generously with salt and pepper.

4 In a large bowl, place onion, carrot, pumpkin, zucchini and remaining olive oil. Toss to combine and transfer to the baking tray, scattering around the chicken.

5 Roast for 45 minutes, or until chicken is crispy and golden brown on the outside and juices run clear, and the vegetables are cooked. Rest for 10 minutes before serving.

6 Transfer the vegetables to a bowl, toss through rocket and diced avocado, and serve alongside the chicken.

Ⓕ♀ MACROS Cals : 680 CHO : 13g P : 58g Fat : 46g
Ⓜ♂ MACROS Cals : 962 CHO : 16g P : 86g Fat : 63g

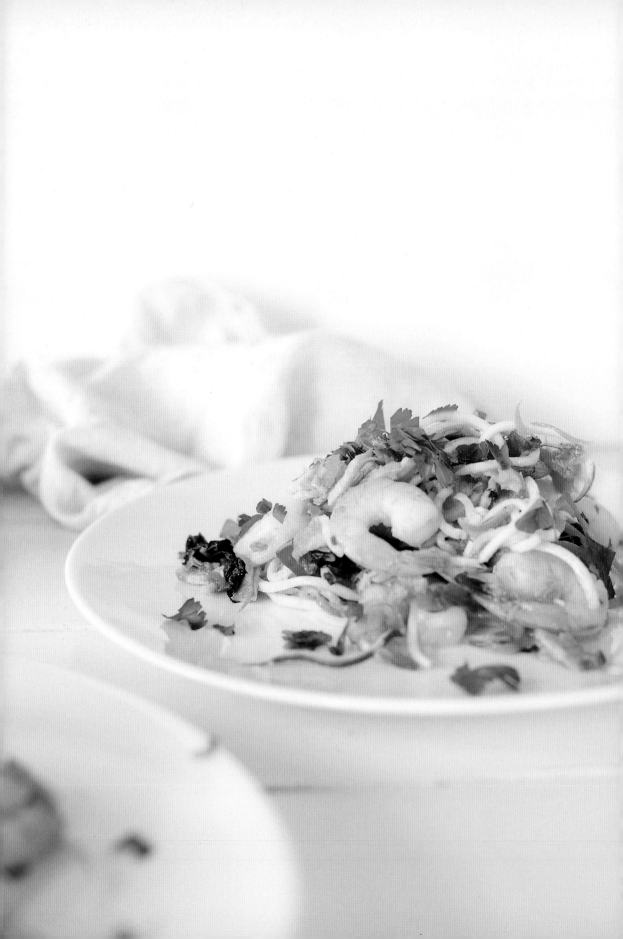

SIMPLE PRAWN 'PASTA'

SERVES ⒡Ⓜ 2   PREP : 10 MINUTES   COOK : 15 MINUTES

With this recipe you will soon learn that carrots, zucchini and squash make great spaghetti substitutes! If you're not a fan of prawns, you can easily make this with chicken or beef.

2 tablespoons cold-pressed extra-virgin coconut oil / 3 tablespoons cold-pressed extra-virgin coconut oil

½ onion, finely chopped / 1 onion, finely chopped

2 cloves garlic, crushed

1 red chilli, deseeded and finely chopped

4 rashers pasture-raised bacon, diced

1 carrot, spiralised

300g green prawns, peeled and deveined / 350g green prawns, peeled and deveined

20g Tuscan kale, roughly chopped

2 zucchinis, spiralised

1 squash, spiralised

¼ bunch parsley, roughly chopped

sea salt and pepper, to taste

1 Heat 1 tablespoon of the coconut oil in a frypan over medium heat and sauté onion, garlic, chilli and bacon for 2–3 minutes, or until golden.

2 Add carrot noodles and quickly sauté until softened.

3 Add remaining oil and prawns, and toss until prawns are cooked through.

4 Add kale, zucchini and squash, and sauté until kale is wilted and noodles are softened.

5 Stir through parsley, season well with salt and pepper, and serve.

Ⓕ MACROS Cals : **429** CHO : **10g** P : **44g** Fat : **20g**
Ⓜ MACROS Cals : **498** CHO : **11g** P : **51g** Fat : **30g**

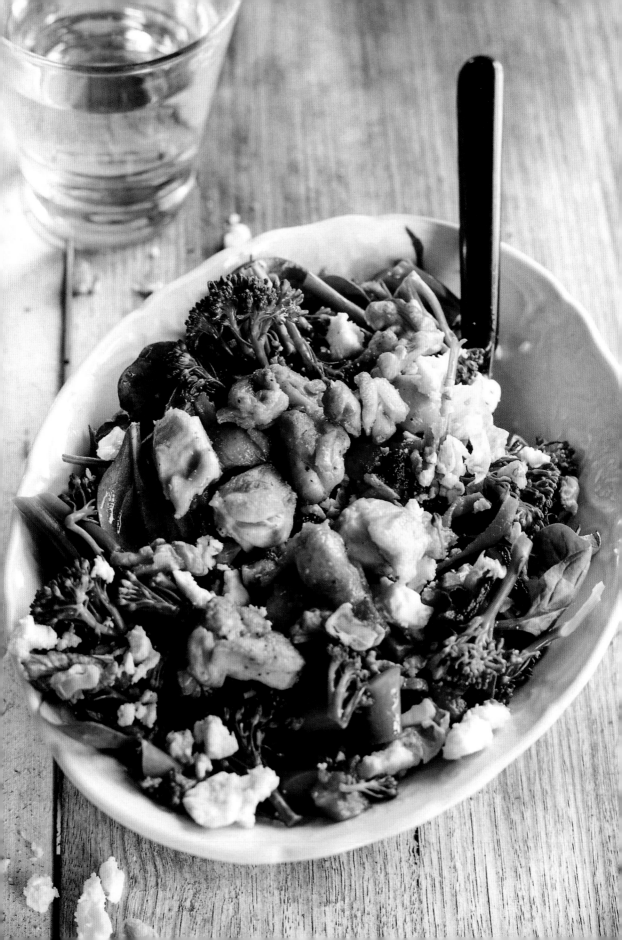

PUMPKIN & FETA CHICKEN SALAD

SERVES Ⓕ ♂ 2   PREP : 10 MINUTES   COOK : 20 MINUTES

This salad is another regular in my household. I've mentioned how much I adore pumpkin roasted with coconut oil and salt, and it's also one of my favourite salad additions. While I prefer to roast my pumpkin on a Sunday to save time mid-week, nothing beats it fresh out of the oven when you do have more time to dedicate to meal prep.

1 cup diced pumpkin

2 tablespoons cold-pressed extra-virgin coconut oil / ¼ cup cold-pressed extra-virgin coconut oil

1 bunch broccolini

200g free-range chicken thigh fillets / 300g free-range chicken thigh fillets

sea salt and pepper, to taste

20g spinach leaves / 50g spinach leaves

1 tablespoon kimchi or sauerkraut

30g goat's feta

30g walnuts, chopped

2 tablespoons extra-virgin olive oil

2 tablespoons apple cider vinegar

1   Preheat oven to 180°C and line a baking tray with baking paper.

2   In a large bowl, toss diced pumpkin in half the coconut oil, transfer to the baking tray and bake for 15 minutes, or until soft.

3   Meanwhile, bring a small saucepan of water to the boil. Place broccolini in a colander or steamer basket, cover with a lid and steam for 4–5 minutes. Remove from the colander or steamer basket and set aside to cool.

4   Heat a frypan over medium heat and add the remaining coconut oil. Season chicken with salt and pepper and add to the pan, cooking for 2–3 minutes each side. Remove from pan, allow to cool slightly then dice the chicken.

5   Place spinach in a large bowl or plate. Add fermented vegetables, roasted pumpkin and steamed broccolini. Crumble feta on top and sprinkle with walnuts.

6   Combine oil with vinegar and toss through salad. Top with diced chicken.

Ⓕ MACROS Cals : 520 CHO : 9g P : 27g Fat : 43g
♂ MACROS Cals : 650 CHO : 9g P : 27g Fat : 57g

CHICKEN ABUNDANCE BOWL #1

SERVES (F) (M) 2   PREP : 10 MINUTES   COOK : 20 MINUTES

½ cup diced pumpkin
1½ tablespoons extra-virgin
   olive oil
¼ teaspoon cinnamon
sea salt and pepper, to taste
300g free-range chicken breast
   fillet
1 cos lettuce, roughly torn
125g cherry tomatoes,
   quartered
1 zucchini, spiralised
1 carrot, spiralised
1 baby beetroot, spiralised
1 red capsicum, sliced
1 avocado, mashed
50g goat's feta
2 tablespoons pumpkin seeds

1 Preheat oven to 180°C and line a baking tray with
   baking paper.

2 In a large bowl, toss diced pumpkin with ½ tablespoon
   of the olive oil and the cinnamon, and season well with
   salt and pepper. Transfer to the baking tray and bake for
   15 minutes, or until soft and lightly brown.

3 In an oiled frypan over medium–high heat, or on a hot
   barbecue plate, grill chicken for 3–5 minutes each side.
   Rest for 1 minute and slice.

4 To serve, place lettuce at the bottom of each bowl. Add
   cherry tomatoes, pumpkin, zucchini, carrot, beetroot and
   capsicum in piles next to each other. Top with chicken,
   avocado and feta. Scatter pumpkin seeds on top, season
   well with salt and pepper, and drizzle with remaining oil.

(F) MACROS Cals : 580 CHO : 24g P : 44g Fat : 37g
(M) MACROS Cals : 580 CHO : 24g P : 44g Fat : 37g

CHICKEN ABUNDANCE BOWL #2

SERVES (F) (M) 2   PREP : 10 MINUTES   COOK : 15 MINUTES

1 corn cob
8 florets of broccoli
½ teaspoon cold-pressed extra-
   virgin coconut oil
100g haloumi, cut into 5cm strips
200g free-range chicken thigh
   fillets, diced / 300g free-range
   chicken thigh fillets, diced
2 zucchinis, spiralised
2 carrots, spiralised
250g cherry tomatoes, quartered
1 cos lettuce, roughly chopped
½ avocado, roughly mashed
2 tablespoons roughly chopped
   coriander
1 lime, halved
sea salt and pepper, to taste
1 tablespoon extra-virgin
   olive oil

1 Bring a small saucepan of water to the boil. Place corn and
   broccoli in a colander or steamer basket, cover with a lid
   and steam for 4–5 minutes. Remove from the colander or
   steamer basket and set aside. Once cooled, remove corn
   kernels from the cob.

2 Heat a frypan over medium heat and melt the coconut oil.
   Fry haloumi for 2 minutes on each side, or until golden.
   Set aside.

3 Add chicken to pan and sauté for 4 minutes, or until golden.

4 Take two bowls and place the chicken in the middle of
   each bowl. Place the remaining ingredients in the bowl
   in segments – zucchini and carrot noodles, corn kernels,
   broccoli, cherry tomatoes, lettuce, haloumi and mashed
   avocado. Top with coriander and a squeeze of lime. Season
   well with salt and pepper and drizzle with olive oil.

(F) MACROS Cals : 615 CHO : 38g P : 49g Fat : 34g
(M) MACROS Cals : 778 CHO : 42g P : 66g Fat : 43g

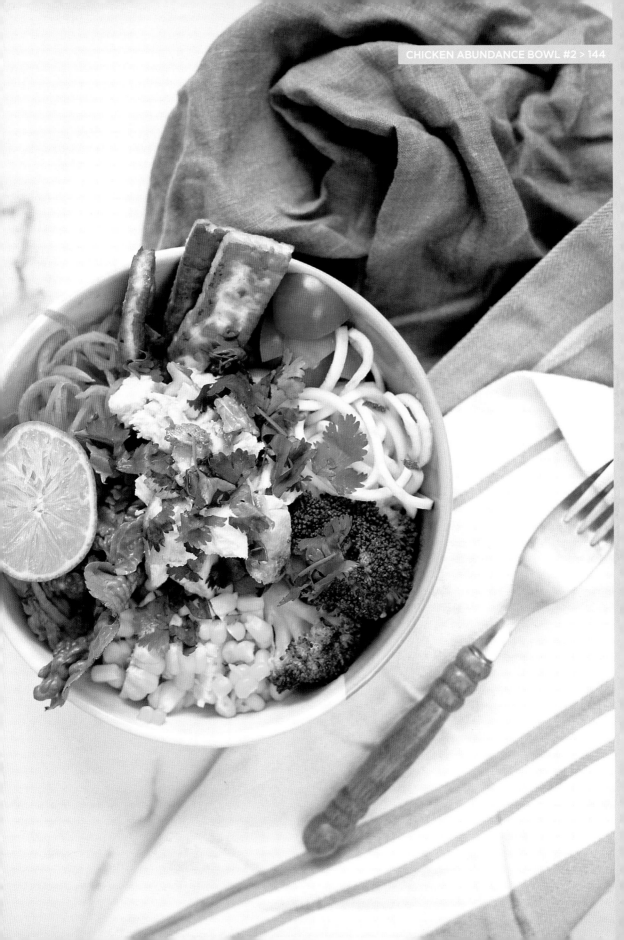

VEGIE ABUNDANCE BOWL

SERVES Ⓕ Ⓜ 2   PREP : 10 MINUTES   COOK : 35 MINUTES

I've shown you two variations of a Chicken Abundance Bowl and this vegetarian version is just as good. The Avocado Dressing is heavenly, and the addition of kimchi makes it very good for your gut health.

sweet potato, cut into discs (about 1 cup)
½ head of broccoli, cut into florets
1 teaspoon cold-pressed extra-virgin coconut oil
½ teaspoon chilli flakes
sea salt and pepper, to taste
1 red capsicum, sliced
2 carrots, spiralised
10 snow peas, trimmed
2 cups spinach leaves
2 tablespoons kimchi
2 tablespoons pumpkin seeds

AVOCADO DRESSING
½ avocado
⅓ cup extra-virgin olive oil
1 lime, juiced
½ teaspoon garlic powder
½ bunch basil
sea salt and pepper, to taste

1 Preheat oven to 180°C and line a baking tray with baking paper.

2 In a large bowl, toss sweet potato discs and broccoli florets in coconut oil and chilli flakes, and season well with salt and pepper. Transfer sweet potato only to the baking tray and bake for 10 minutes. At the 10-minute mark, turn the sweet potato and add broccoli. Bake for a further 10 minutes, or until both have softened and are golden.

3 To make the Avocado Dressing, place all the dressing ingredients in a blender or food processor and blitz until smooth and creamy. Blend in a little water if you prefer a thinner dressing.

4 Take two bowls and place sweet potato discs on the side of each bowl. Next, add broccoli, then capsicum slices, spiralised carrot, snow peas, spinach and kimchi in segments. Scatter pumpkin seeds over the top and drizzle with avocado dressing.

Ⓕ MACROS Cals : **659** CHO : **35g** P : **17g** Fat : **57g**
Ⓜ MACROS Cals : **659** CHO : **35g** P : **17g** Fat : **57g**

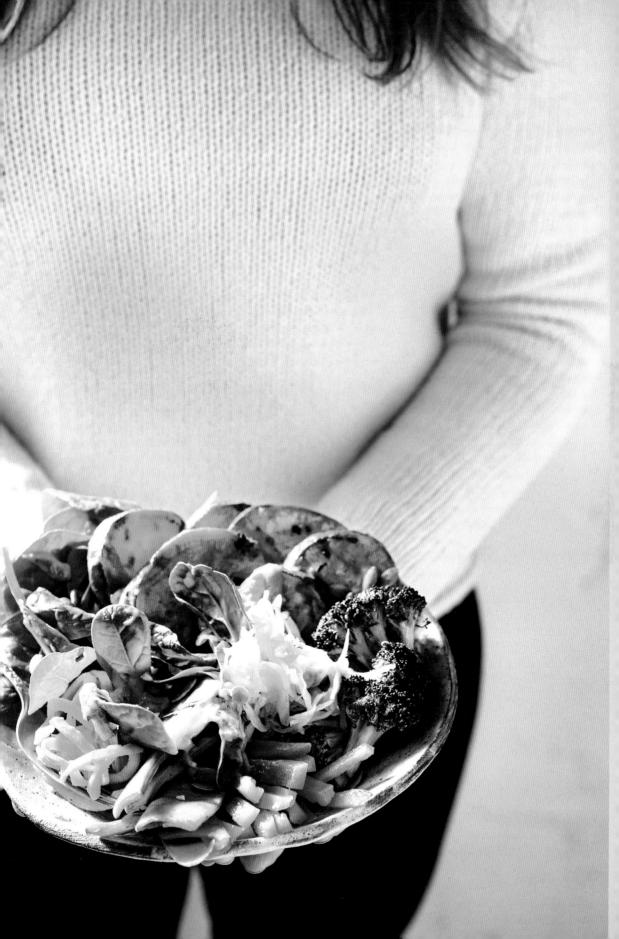

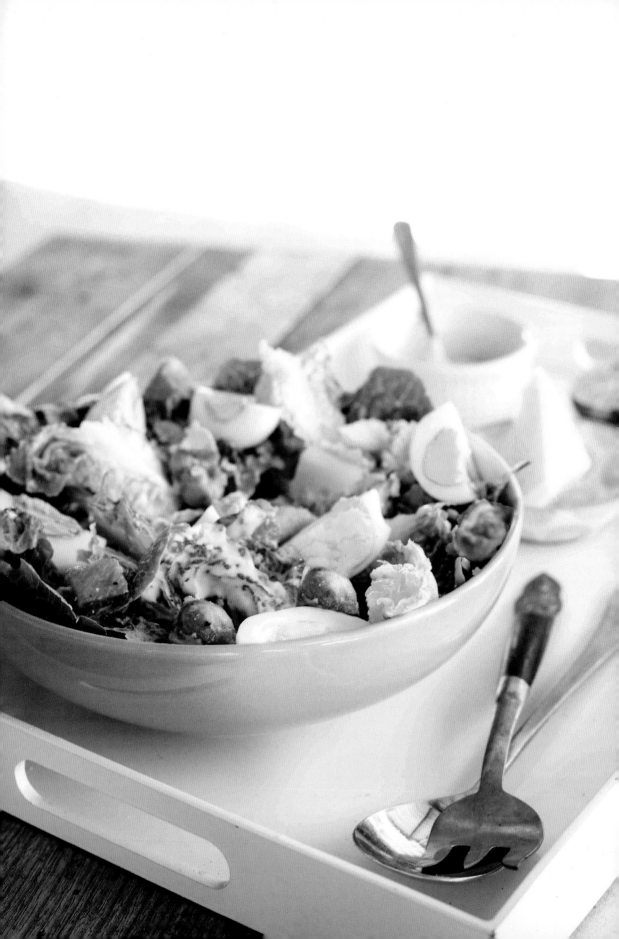

CHICKEN CAESAR SALAD

SERVES (F) (M) 2   PREP : 10 MINUTES   COOK : 15 MINUTES

You are going to absolutely love my take on a chicken caesar salad! The gluten-free bread is optional but it's a lovely treat when you want to closely replicate a more traditional version. Per serve there is still only 12g of carbohydrates, so it definitely fits our LCHF template.

2 free-range eggs
1 slice gluten-free bread,
    roughly torn, optional
1 tablespoon grass-fed butter
4 rashers pasture-raised
    bacon, diced
2 free-range chicken thigh
    fillets, diced
sea salt and pepper, to taste
2 heads of baby cos lettuce,
    roughly torn
2 tablespoons grated parmesan
    cheese
anchovies, for serving, optional

DRESSING
1 large egg, free range
1 lime, zested and juiced
1 tablespoon apple cider
    vinegar
1 teaspoon Dijon mustard
2 anchovies, plus extra, optional
¼ teaspoon sea salt
¾ cup macadamia oil

1   To boil eggs: Bring a small saucepan of water to the boil. Carefully add eggs and reduce heat to a simmer. Cook for 4–5 minutes. Run under cold water before peeling and cutting in quarters.

2   If making bread croutons: Preheat oven to 180°C and line a baking tray with baking paper. Place torn bread on the tray and bake for 5–7 minutes, or until golden.

3   Heat a medium frypan over medium heat, add butter and bacon and fry for 2 minutes. Add chicken, season well with salt and pepper and cook for 5–7 minutes, or until golden and cooked through.

4   To make the dressing: In a tall glass jar, place egg, lime zest and juice, vinegar, mustard, anchovies and sea salt. Add oil and allow to sit for a minute. Insert a stick blender and blend for 1 minute, or until desired thickness achieved.

5   In a large bowl, combine cos lettuce, chicken, bacon, quartered eggs and croutons. Stir through 1–2 tablespoons of the dressing and mix well to combine. Sprinkle parmesan on top and add an extra anchovy or two if desired. Any remaining dressing can be stored in the fridge for up to 7 days.

(F)   MACROS   Cals : **595**   CHO : **12g**   P : **23g**   Fat : **49g**
(M)   MACROS   Cals : **595**   CHO : **12g**   P : **23g**   Fat : **49g**

SALMON WITH GREEN SALAD

SERVES Ⓕ Ⓜ 2   PREP : 10 MINUTES   COOK : 10 MINUTES

40g rocket leaves /
  60g rocket leaves
125g cherry tomatoes,
  quartered
1 avocado, diced
2 tablespoons roughly
  chopped walnuts
2 tablespoons kimchi
½ lemon
1 tablespoon cold-pressed
  extra-virgin coconut oil
2 × 120g salmon fillets,
  preferably wild caught /
  2 × 150g salmon fillets,
  preferably wild caught
sea salt, to taste

1   In a large bowl, place rocket, cherry tomatoes, avocado, walnuts and kimchi, and toss to combine. Squeeze lemon over salad and divide between two plates.

2   Heat coconut oil in a medium frypan and add salmon fillets, skin side down. Season with salt and cook for 5 minutes over medium–high heat, or until skin is crispy, then flip the salmon and continue cooking the other side to your liking.

3   Serve salmon alongside green salad and enjoy.

Ⓕ   MACROS   Cals : **498**   CHO : **11g**   P : **33g**   Fat : **37g**
Ⓜ   MACROS   Cals : **618**   CHO : **11g**   P : **47g**   Fat : **43g**

BARBECUED PRAWN SALAD

SERVES Ⓕ Ⓜ 2   PREP : 10 MINUTES + 20 MINUTES MARINATING   COOK : 5 MINUTES

This is one of my favourite summer meals and a really simple one to serve when you have friends over for dinner. If you marinate the prawns ahead of time, cooking them is super-quick and easy, which means you'll have more time to spend with your guests.

1 red chilli, deseeded and
  finely chopped
1 garlic clove, finely chopped
1 lemon, zested and juiced
¼ cup extra-virgin olive oil
300g green prawns, peeled
  and deveined
½ head of iceberg lettuce,
  roughly chopped
2 celery stalks, diced
125g cherry tomatoes,
  quartered
1 avocado, diced
1 tablespoon finely chopped
  chives
1 tablespoon sunflower seeds /
  2 tablespoons sunflower seeds
sea salt and pepper, to taste

1   Combine chilli, garlic, lemon zest, half the lemon juice and olive oil in a bowl. Marinate prawns for 20 minutes.

2   In a large salad bowl, combine lettuce, celery, tomatoes, avocado, chives and sunflower seeds.

3   Heat a barbecue grill plate to high and cook prawns for 2–4 minutes each side, or until cooked through.

4   Toss prawns through the salad and pour the remaining lemon juice over the top. Season if required.

Ⓕ   MACROS   Cals : **561**   CHO : **13g**   P : **35g**   Fat : **42g**
Ⓜ   MACROS   Cals : **586**   CHO : **14g**   P : **36g**   Fat : **45g**

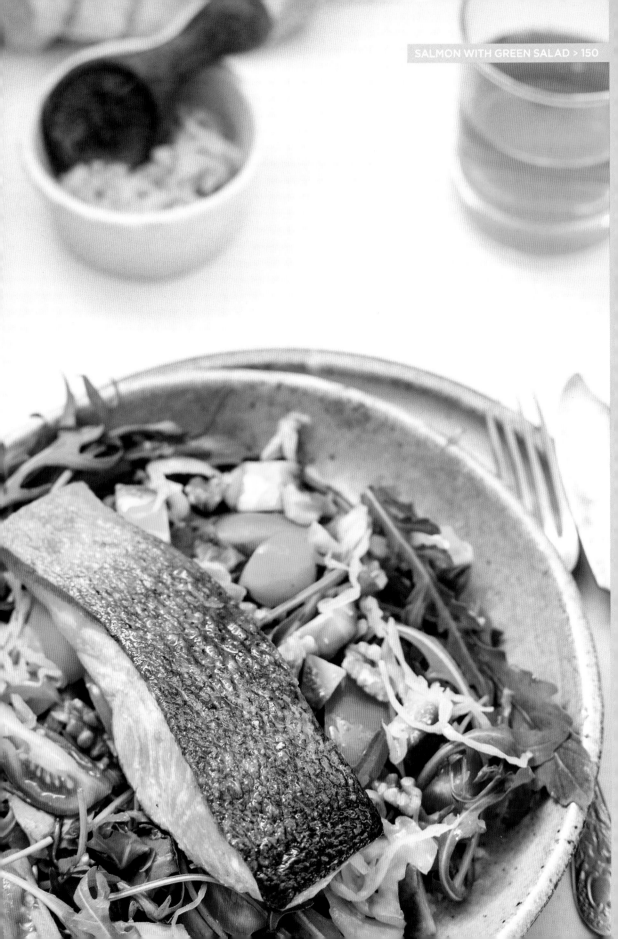

BARBECUED PRAWN SALAD > 150

LAMB & CAULIFLOWER SALAD > 153

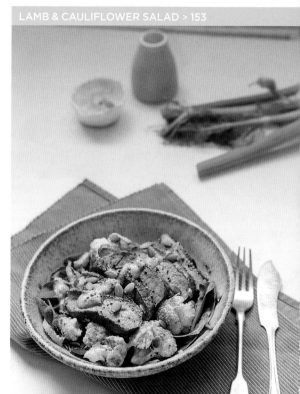

GREEN VEGIE SLICE > 153

CHICKEN 'PASTA' WITH CASHEW PESTO > 154

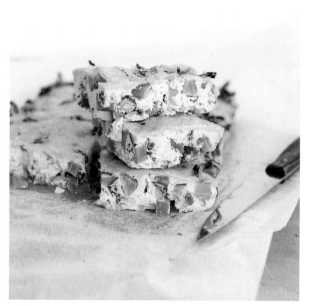

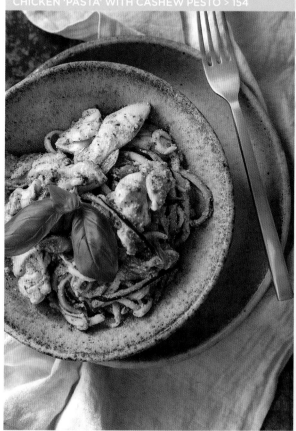

LAMB & CAULIFLOWER SALAD

SERVES Ⓕ Ⓜ 4 / 2   PREP : 10 MINUTES   COOK : 30 MINUTES

Roasted cauliflower, barbecued lamb and the most delicious almond butter dressing – you'll wonder where this meal has been all your life!

¼ cup cold-pressed extra-virgin coconut oil, melted
1 tablespoon cumin
1 tablespoon paprika
1 teaspoon garlic powder
1 teaspoon sea salt
1 head of cauliflower, cut into florets
1 fennel bulb, quartered
400g lamb fillets /
    300g lamb fillets
1 tablespoon extra-virgin olive oil
40g spinach leaves
¼ cup pumpkin seeds
sea salt and pepper, to taste

DRESSING
2 tablespoons almond butter
1 lemon, juiced
2 tablespoons extra-virgin olive oil
¼ teaspoon sea salt

1 Preheat oven to 180°C and line a baking tray with baking paper.

2 In a large bowl, combine coconut oil, cumin, paprika, garlic powder and sea salt. Toss cauliflower and fennel in the spices until well coated. Place on the baking tray and roast in the oven for 20 minutes. Turn, and continue to roast for another 20 minutes or so, until golden brown.

3 To make the dressing, place all the ingredients plus 2 tablespoons of water in a small bowl and whisk to combine. If you desire a thinner consistency, whisk in a little extra water.

4 Heat a barbecue grill on medium–high heat. Brush lamb fillets with olive oil and grill for 6 minutes, turning each minute. Allow to rest for 5 minutes before slicing.

5 In a large bowl, combine roasted cauliflower and fennel with spinach and pumpkin seeds. Stir through dressing, season well with salt and pepper, and top with sliced lamb.

Ⓕ MACROS Cals : **452** CHO : **19g** P : **37g** Fat : **40g**
Ⓜ MACROS Cals : **837** CHO : **37g** P : **60g** Fat : **77g**

GREEN VEGIE SLICE

SERVES Ⓕ Ⓜ 6 / 4   PREP : 10 MINUTES   COOK : 30 MINUTES

¼ cup cold-pressed extra-virgin coconut oil
1 zucchini, finely chopped
½ bunch broccolini, finely chopped
5 free-range eggs
1 cup almond or macadamia nut flour
sea salt and pepper, to taste

1 Preheat oven to 180°C. Grease a quiche tin or baking pan with 1 teaspoon of the coconut oil.

2 Place vegies in a large bowl. Whisk eggs in a separate bowl then add to vegies with remaining oil and flour. Stir well and season with salt and pepper to taste.

3 Pour into the quiche tin or pan and bake for 20–30 minutes, or until cooked through.

4 Allow to cool before slicing. Delicious warm or cold, the slice will keep in the fridge for 4–5 days.

Ⓕ MACROS Cals : **397** CHO : **5g** P : **8g** Fat : **39g**
Ⓜ MACROS Cals : **595** CHO : **7g** P : **14g** Fat : **59g**

CHICKEN 'PASTA' WITH CASHEW PESTO

SERVES (F) (M) 2   PREP : 10 MINUTES   COOK : 10 MINUTES

This recipe is so fresh, nutrient-dense and delicious, you really won't miss the carbs.
It serves two, but if you enjoy this as much as I do, you'll want to double this recipe.

1 tablespoon cold-pressed
   extra-virgin coconut oil
1 garlic clove, crushed
1 chilli, deseeded and finely
   chopped
300g free-range chicken thigh
   fillets, diced
125g cherry tomatoes
3 zucchinis, spiralised
sea salt and pepper to taste
2 basil leaves, for serving

PESTO
¾ cup raw cashews, soaked
   for 4–6 hours then drained
1 cup fresh basil leaves
½ cup extra-virgin olive oil
2 heaped tablespoons
   nutritional yeast
½ lemon, juiced (or more to taste)

1. To make the pesto, place all the pesto ingredients in a food processor or blender and blend until combined and smooth. Reserve 2–3 tablespoons and store the rest in an airtight glass container in the fridge for 5–7 days.

2. Melt the coconut oil in a frypan over medium heat, add garlic and chilli and sauté for 1 minute, or until fragrant.

3. Add chicken and sauté for 4 minutes, or until golden and cooked through.

4. Add cherry tomatoes and 2 tablespoons of the pesto, and stir through.

5. Add zucchini noodles and sauté for 3–4 minutes. Season well with salt and pepper.

6. Serve the noodles with a dollop of the reserved pesto and a fresh basil leaf.

(F) MACROS Cals : **656** CHO : **15g** P : **40g** Fat : **41g**
(M) MACROS Cals : **656** CHO : **15g** P : **40g** Fat : **41g**

VEGETABLE COCONUT CURRY

SERVES (F) (M) 3 / 2   PREP : 10 MINUTES   COOK : 40 MINUTES

1 tablespoon cold-pressed
   extra-virgin coconut oil
1 red onion, diced
1 red chilli, deseeded and
   finely chopped
300g organic tempeh, cut into
   1–2cm cubes
3 garlic cloves, crushed
1 red capsicum, diced
10 button mushrooms, sliced
2 zucchinis, diced
1 head of broccoli, cut into florets
3 teaspoons curry powder
2 teaspoons vegetable stock
1 cup coconut cream
sea salt and pepper, to taste

1. Heat coconut oil in a large frypan over high heat, add onion and chilli, and sauté for 1–2 minutes, or until the onion has softened.

2. Add tempeh and garlic and sauté for 1–2 minutes, or until the tempeh has browned.

3. Stir in vegetables, curry powder, vegetable stock and coconut cream. Bring to the boil then reduce heat and simmer for 30 minutes. Season well with salt and pepper before serving.

(F) MACROS Cals : **339** CHO : **25g** P : **23g** Fat : **18g**
(M) MACROS Cals : **508** CHO : **38g** P : **34g** Fat : **27g**

I wanted to show how to cook tempeh, as people often screw their nose up at it simply because they haven't experienced how good it can be. Use what you learn in this recipe to replace chicken, fish, beef or lamb in any curry or stir-fry for the days when you feel like lowering your animal protein intake.

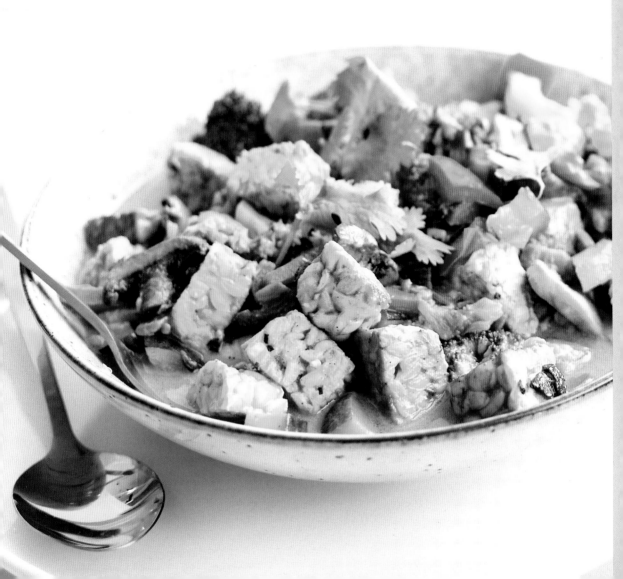

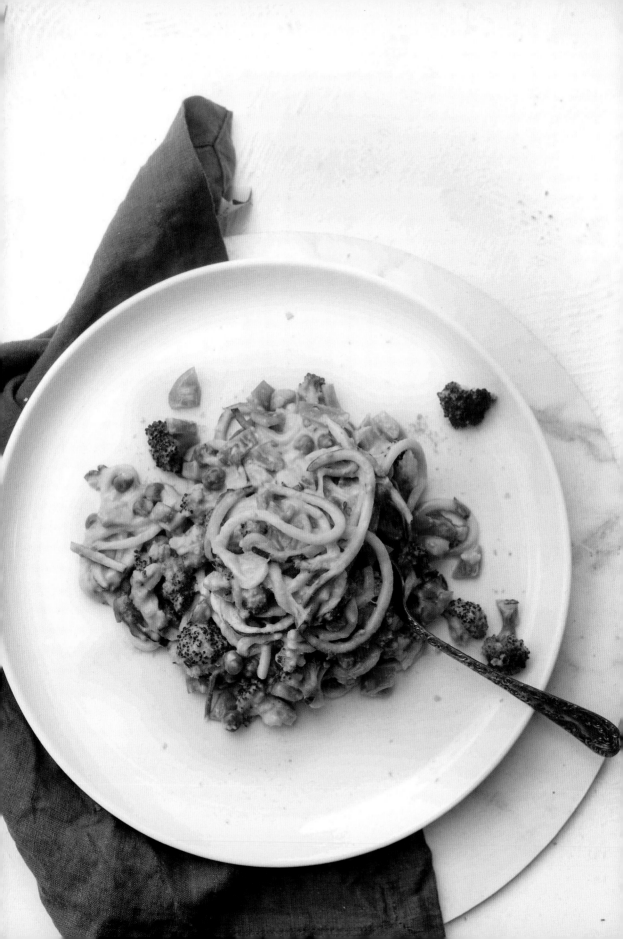

GREEN LCHF 'PASTA'

SERVES (F) (M) 2   PREP : 10 MINUTES   COOK : 15 MINUTES

½ head of broccoli, cut into small florets / 1 head of broccoli, cut into small florets

½ cup frozen peas

½ tablespoon cold-pressed extra-virgin coconut oil

3 zucchinis, spiralised / 4 zucchinis, spiralised

125g cherry tomatoes, quartered

sea salt and pepper

1 teaspoon nutritional yeast

AVOCADO & TAHINI DRESSING

½ avocado / 1 avocado

½ tablespoon tahini / 1 tablespoon tahini

½ tablespoon extra-virgin olive oil / 1 tablespoon extra-virgin olive oil

½ bunch basil

1 garlic clove, crushed

1 lemon, juiced

1 To make the Avocado & Tahini Dressing, place all the dressing ingredients in a blender or food processor and blitz until smooth and creamy. Blend in a little water if you prefer a thinner dressing.

2 Bring a small saucepan of water to the boil. Place broccoli and peas in a colander or steamer basket, cover with a lid and steam for 4–5 minutes. Transfer to a large bowl.

3 Melt coconut oil in a frypan over medium heat, add zucchini noodles and sauté for 3–4 minutes.

4 Add zucchini noodles and cherry tomatoes to the bowl of broccoli and peas. Stir through dressing, season well with salt and pepper, and serve topped with nutritional yeast.

(F) MACROS Cals : **258**   CHO : **22g**   P : **10g**   Fat : **16g**
(M) MACROS Cals : **432**   CHO : **36g**   P : **16g**   Fat : **28g**

MUSHROOM BURGERS WITH KALE CHIPS

SERVES Ⓕ Ⓜ 2 / 1   PREP : 10 MINUTES   COOK : 15 MINUTES

Portobello mushrooms are a delicious and nutrient-dense bread substitute, and these burgers are on the table in less than 20 minutes. I love to add Kale Chips (see below) for a Friday- or Saturday-night meal. If you're yet to try kale chips, you're in for a treat!

4 portobello mushrooms /
  2 portobello mushrooms
1 teaspoon fresh thyme leaves
75g goat's feta / 50g goat's
  feta
2 rashers pasture-raised
  bacon, grilled
2 free-range eggs, fried /
  1 free-range egg, fried
½ tomato, sliced
1 avocado, mashed
1 beetroot, grated
½ carrot, grated
20g rocket leaves
sea salt and pepper, to taste

KALE CHIPS
1 small bunch kale
2 tablespoons cold-pressed
  extra-virgin coconut oil
sea salt, to taste

1 To make the kale chips, preheat the oven to 120°C and line a baking tray with baking paper. Roughly tear the kale leaves from the stems and wash and dry thoroughly.

2 Add kale leaves to the baking tray, toss with coconut oil and salt and bake for 5–10 minutes, or until lightly browned on top. Be sure to check them regularly as they do cook fast!

3 Line another baking tray with baking paper and place mushrooms on the tray. Place thyme and feta on top of 2 mushrooms (or 1 mushroom, if making a single serve). Bake for 8–10 minutes, or until feta starts to melt.

4 Remove the mushrooms from the oven. On top of the melted feta, place bacon, eggs, tomato, avocado, beetroot, carrot and rocket. Season well with salt and pepper and top with another mushroom.

5 Serve with kale chips and enjoy.

Ⓕ MACROS Cals : 579   CHO : 29g   P : 27g   Fat : 42g
Ⓜ MACROS Cals : 791   CHO : 44g   P : 34g   Fat : 58g

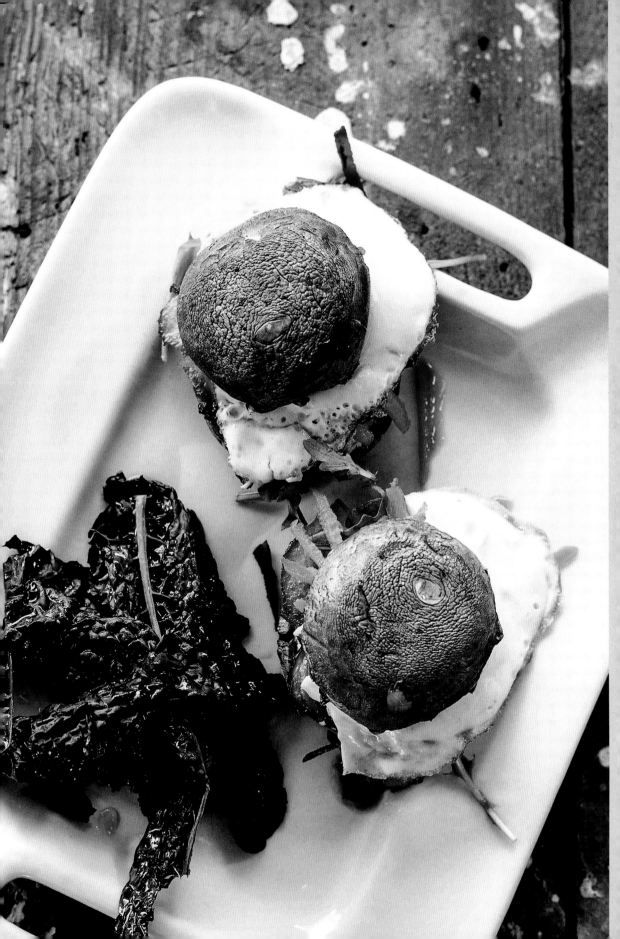

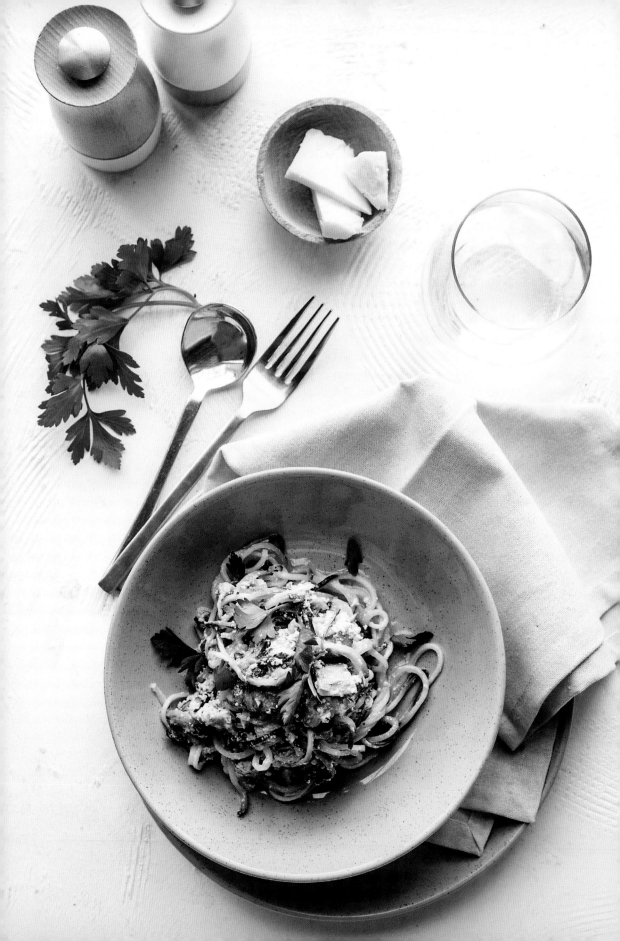

ZUCCHINI CARBONARA

SERVES Ⓕ Ⓜ 4 / 2   PREP : 5 MINUTES   COOK : 10 MINUTES

3 tablespoons grass-fed butter
4 rashers pasture-raised bacon,
  roughly chopped
½ red onion, finely diced
1 garlic clove, crushed
2 free-range eggs
½ cup coconut milk
¼ cup grated parmesan
2 tablespoons capers, drained
2 tablespoons roughly chopped
  parsley
4 zucchinis, spiralised
sea salt and pepper, to taste

1 Heat a frypan over medium heat and add half the butter.
   Add the bacon, onion and garlic and fry for 4–6 minutes,
   or until golden. Remove from the pan and set aside.

2 In a small bowl, whisk together the eggs, coconut milk,
   parmesan, capers and parsley. Season well and set aside.

3 Return the frypan to medium heat and add the remaining
   butter. Add the zucchini noodles and sauté for 1 minute.
   Return the bacon mixture to the pan.

4 Reduce the heat to low and slowly pour the egg and milk
   mixture into the pan. Stir the mixture in quickly so it forms
   a sauce, rather than a scramble! Season well and serve
   immediately, topping with additional parsley if desired.

Ⓕ MACROS Cals : 324 CHO : 9g   P : 18g Fat : 23g
Ⓜ MACROS Cals : 648 CHO : 18g P : 36g Fat : 46g

MIX & MATCH

Here I want to teach you how to create variety in your kitchen by pairing simple proteins with the perfect side dish or two. Real food can be simple, affordable and delicious.

SHEPHERD'S PIE WITH PUMPKIN MASH & BUTTERED GREENS

SERVES ⓕ Ⓜ 6 / 4   PREP : 25 MINUTES   COOK : 25 MINUTES

1 tablespoon cold-pressed extra-virgin coconut oil
2 garlic cloves, chopped
500g grass-fed beef mince /
  600g grass-fed beef mince
400g tomato passata (100% tomatoes)
2 tablespoons tomato paste (no salt added)
1 teaspoon chilli flakes
1 teaspoon cinnamon
1 teaspoon nutmeg
1 carrot, grated
1 zucchini, grated

PUMPKIN MASH

1 small pumpkin, peeled and cut into small pieces
¼ cup grass-fed butter
sea salt and pepper, to taste

BUTTERED GREENS

4 cups roughly chopped broccolini
4 cups diced zucchini
120g grass-fed butter
sea salt, to taste

1 Preheat the oven to 220°C.

2 Heat coconut oil in a large pan over medium heat and sauté garlic until golden brown.

3 Add mince and cook for 15 minutes, stirring to remove any lumps.

4 Add tomato passata, tomato paste and spices, and cook over low heat until the excess liquid evaporates.

5 To make Pumpkin Mash: While the mince mixture is cooking, bring a small saucepan of water to the boil. Place pumpkin in a colander or steamer basket, cover with a lid and steam for 4–5 minutes. Remove from the colander or steamer basket and return to the drained saucepan. Mash with butter and season well with salt and pepper.

6 Stir grated vegetables into the mince mixture and transfer to an 18cm baking dish. Gently spoon the pumpkin mash over the top and press firmly until even. Bake for 20 minutes then finish under the grill so the top is crispy and brown.

7 To make Buttered Greens: While the pie is baking, bring a small saucepan of water to the boil. Place broccolini and zucchini in a colander or steamer basket, cover with a lid and steam for 4–5 minutes. Toss steamed greens with butter and season well with salt.

8 Serve greens alongside shepherd's pie.

ⓕ MACROS Cals : **613**   CHO : **25g**   P : **34g**   Fat : **42g**
Ⓜ MACROS Cals : **775**   CHO : **30g**   P : **36g**   Fat : **59g**

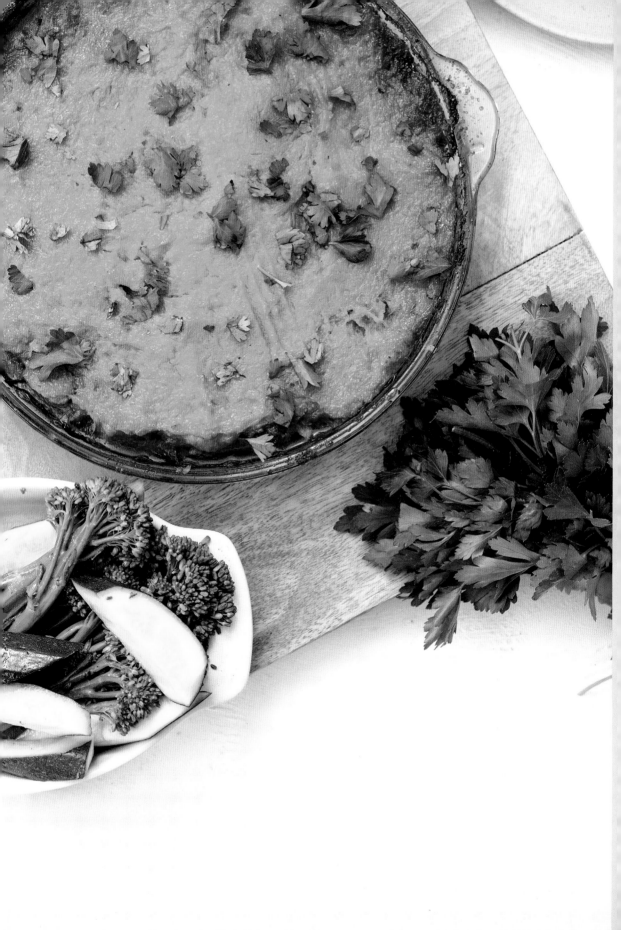

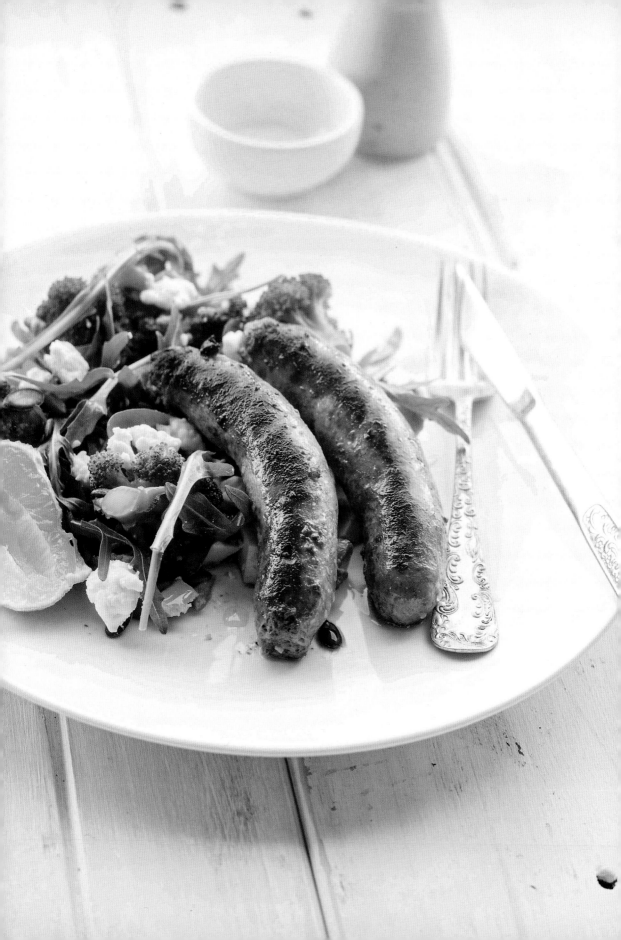

CLEAN SNAGS WITH WARM BROCCOLI SALAD

SERVES Ⓕ Ⓜ 4   PREP : 10 MINUTES   COOK : 10 MINUTES

2 heads of broccoli, cut
  into florets
50g rocket leaves
1 avocado, diced
¼ cup pumpkin seeds
2 tablespoons extra-virgin
  olive oil
½ lemon, juiced
sea salt, to taste
30g goat's feta
8 grass-fed sausages

1 Bring a small saucepan of water to the boil. Place broccoli in a colander or steamer basket, cover with a lid and lightly steam for 4–5 minutes. Remove from the colander or steamer basket.

2 Combine broccoli, rocket, avocado and pumpkin seeds in a large bowl.

3 In a small bowl, whisk together olive oil, lemon juice and salt. Toss through salad and sprinkle with feta.

4 On a preheated barbecue grill over medium heat, cook sausages slowly, turning every couple of minutes until brown all over and cooked through.

5 Remove sausages from heat and serve with Warm Broccoli Salad.

Ⓕ MACROS Cals : 676   CHO : 30g   P : 47g   Fat : 42g
Ⓜ MACROS Cals : 676   CHO : 30g   P : 47g   Fat : 42g

CLEAN SNAGS WITH SUPER SALAD

SERVES Ⓕ Ⓜ 2   PREP : 15 MINUTES   COOK : 10 MINUTES

4 grass-fed sausages

SUPER SALAD
60g spinach and rocket leaves
40g finely chopped red cabbage
1 carrot, grated
1 raw beetroot, grated
125g cherry tomatoes, halved
¼ bunch coriander, roughly
   chopped
¼ bunch basil, roughly chopped
100g blueberries
1 avocado, diced
1 tablespoon avocado oil
sea salt and pepper, to taste
¼ cup pumpkin seeds
50g goat's feta

1 To make Super Salad: In a large bowl, combine all the vegetables, herbs, blueberries and avocado. Add avocado oil and toss gently to combine. Season well with salt and pepper, and top with pumpkin seeds and feta.

2 On a preheated barbecue grill over medium heat, cook sausages slowly, turning every couple of minutes until they are brown all over and cooked through.

3 Remove sausages from heat and serve with the salad.

Ⓕ MACROS Cals : **846** CHO : **33g** P : **51g** Fat : **57g**
Ⓜ MACROS Cals : **846** CHO : **33g** P : **51g** Fat : **57g**

GRASS-FED STEAK WITH SUPER-EASY SIDE SALAD

SERVES Ⓕ Ⓜ 2   PREP : 10 MINUTES + 1–2 HOURS MARINATING   COOK : 10 MINUTES

2 × 120g grass-fed beef eye
   fillet steaks / 2 × 150 grass-fed
   beef eye fillet steaks
2 tablespoons extra-virgin
   olive oil / 4 tablespoons
   extra-virgin olive oil
sea salt and pepper, to taste

SUPER-EASY SIDE SALAD
100g rocket leaves
125g cherry tomatoes, halved
1 avocado, diced
2 tablespoons fermented
   vegetables
2 tablespoons extra-virgin
   olive oil
½ lemon, juiced
sea salt and pepper, to taste

1 Marinate steak in olive oil, sea salt and pepper for 1–2 hours.

2 Drain marinade into a frypan preheated over high heat before adding steak and cooking for 6–8 minutes per side, depending on your desired result. Rest for 5 minutes before serving.

3 To make the side salad: While the steak is cooking, in a large bowl combine rocket, cherry tomatoes, avocado and fermented vegetables. In a small bowl, whisk together olive oil and lemon juice and toss through salad. Season well with salt and pepper.

4 Serve the steak on top of the salad.

Ⓕ MACROS Cals : **604** CHO : **12g** P : **42g** Fat : **46g**
Ⓜ MACROS Cals : **777** CHO : **12g** P : **52g** Fat : **62g**

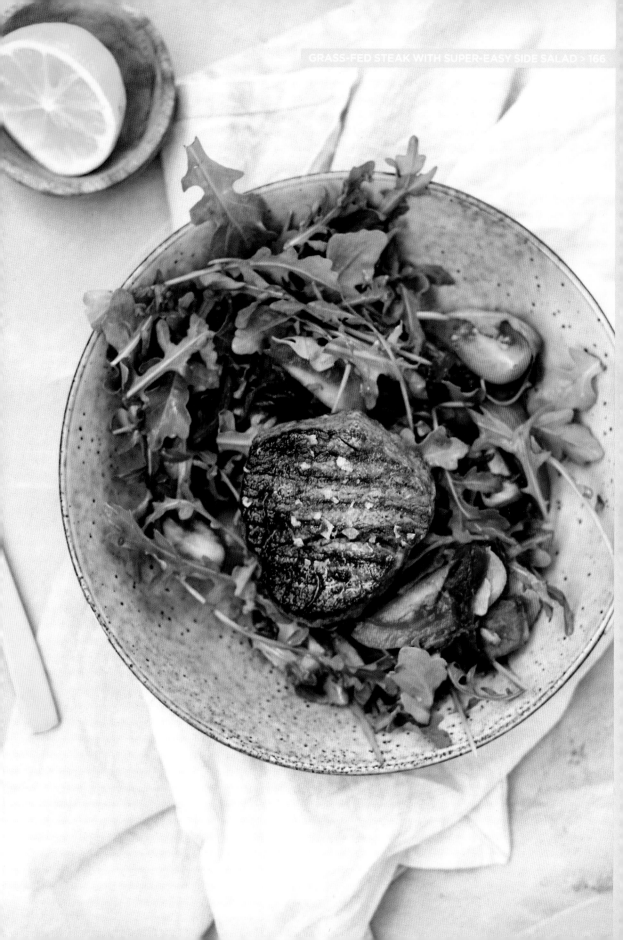

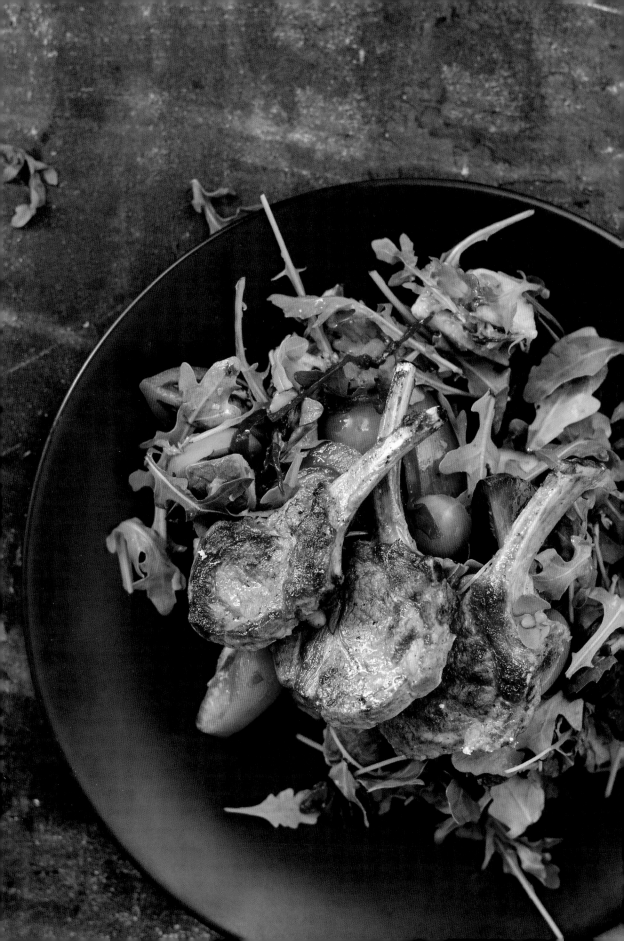

LAMB CUTLETS WITH SUPER-EASY SIDE SALAD

SERVES (F) (M) 2   PREP : 10 MINUTES + 1–2 HOURS MARINATING   COOK : 10 MINUTES

6 grass-fed lamb cutlets /
   8 grass-fed lamb cutlets
¼ cup extra-virgin olive oil
sea salt and pepper, to taste

SUPER-EASY SIDE SALAD
100g rocket leaves
125g cherry tomatoes, halved
1 avocado, diced
2 tablespoons fermented
   vegetables
2 tablespoons extra-virgin
   olive oil
½ lemon, juiced
sea salt and pepper, to taste

1 Marinate lamb cutlets in oil, sea salt and pepper for
   1–2 hours.

2 Drain marinade into a frypan preheated over medium–high
   heat before adding cutlets and cooking on both sides for
   4–6 minutes, or to your liking. Rest for 5 minutes before
   serving.

3 To make Super-easy Side Salad: While the cutlets are
   cooking, in a large bowl combine rocket, cherry tomatoes,
   avocado and fermented vegetables. In a small bowl, whisk
   together olive oil and lemon juice and toss through salad.
   Season well with salt and pepper.

4 Serve cutlets alongside salad.

(F) MACROS Cals : **675** CHO : **12g** P : **30g** Fat : **61g**
(M) MACROS Cals : **730** CHO : **12g** P : **38g** Fat : **63g**

GRASS-FED STEAK WITH ZUCCHINI CHIPS & CAULIFLOWER MASH

SERVES (F) (M) 2   PREP : 10 MINUTES + 1–2 HOURS MARINATING   COOK : 15 MINUTES

2 × 120g grass-fed beef eye fillet steaks / 2 × 150 grass-fed beef eye fillet steaks
2 tablespoons extra-virgin olive oil / 4 tablespoons extra-virgin olive oil
sea salt and pepper, to taste

ZUCCHINI CHIPS
1 large zucchini, cut into chip-like pieces
2 tablespoons cold-pressed extra-virgin coconut oil
sea salt, to taste

CAULIFLOWER MASH
1 medium head of cauliflower, cut into florets
2 tablespoons grass-fed butter
sea salt, to taste

1 Marinate steak in olive oil, sea salt and pepper for 1–2 hours.

2 To make Zucchini Chips: Preheat oven to 180°C and line a baking tray with baking paper. Toss the zucchini with oil and salt. Bake for 10–15 minutes. Finish off under the grill until crispy. Set aside.

3 Drain marinade into a frypan preheated over high heat before adding steak and cooking for 6–8 minutes per side, depending on your desired result. Rest for 5 minutes before serving.

4 To make Cauliflower Mash: While the steak is cooking, bring a small saucepan of water to the boil. Place cauliflower in a colander or steamer basket, cover with a lid and steam for 4–5 minutes. Remove from the colander or steamer basket and return to drained saucepan. Mash with butter and season with salt to taste.

5 Serve Cauliflower Mash and Zucchini Chips alongside the steak.

(F) MACROS Cals : **600** CHO : **26g** P : **34g** Fat : **43g**
(M) MACROS Cals : **755** CHO : **27g** P : **40g** Fat : **58g**

LAMB CUTLETS WITH SIMPLE GREEK SALAD

SERVES (F) (M) 2   PREP : 10 MINUTES + 1–2 HOURS MARINATING   COOK : 10 MINUTES

6 grass-fed lamb cutlets / 8 grass-fed lamb cutlets
¼ cup extra-virgin olive oil
sea salt and pepper, to taste

SIMPLE GREEK SALAD
½ cos lettuce, leaves roughly torn
100g cherry tomatoes, quartered
½ cucumber, diced
15g goat's feta, crumbled
10 black olives, halved and pitted
2 tablespoons extra-virgin olive oil
1 lemon, juiced
sea salt and pepper, to taste

1 Marinate lamb cutlets in oil, sea salt and pepper for 1–2 hours.

2 Drain marinade into a frypan preheated over medium–high heat before adding cutlets and cooking on both sides for 4–6 minutes, or to your liking. Rest for 5 minutes before serving.

3 To make Greek Salad: While the cutlets are cooking, in a large bowl combine lettuce, cherry tomatoes, cucumber, feta and olives. In a small bowl, whisk together olive oil and lemon juice, and toss through the salad. Season well with salt and pepper.

4 Serve cutlets alongside salad.

(F) MACROS Cals : **577** CHO : **6g** P : **29g** Fat : **52g**
(M) MACROS Cals : **632** CHO : **6g** P : **37g** Fat : **54g**

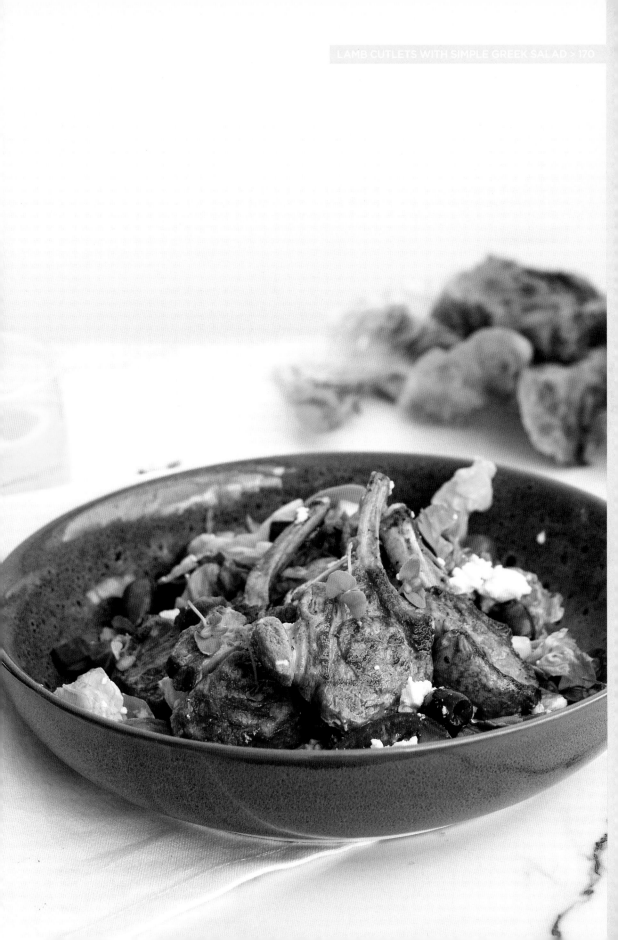

LAMB CUTLETS WITH SUPER SALAD

SERVES Ⓕ Ⓜ 2   PREP : 15 MINUTES + 1–2 HOURS MARINATING   COOK : 10 MINUTES

6 grass-fed lamb cutlets /
 8 grass-fed lamb cutlets
¼ cup extra-virgin olive oil
sea salt and pepper, to taste

SUPER SALAD
60g spinach and rocket leaves
40g finely chopped red cabbage
1 carrot, grated
1 raw beetroot, grated
125g cherry tomatoes, halved
¼ bunch coriander, roughly
   chopped
¼ bunch basil, roughly chopped
100g blueberries
1 avocado, diced
1 tablespoon avocado oil
sea salt and pepper, to taste
¼ cup pumpkin seeds
50g goat's feta

1 Marinate lamb cutlets in oil, sea salt and pepper for
   1–2 hours.

2 Drain marinade into a frypan preheated over medium–high
   heat before adding cutlets and cooking on both sides for
   4–6 minutes, or to your liking. Rest for 5 minutes before
   serving.

3 To make Super Salad: While lamb is cooking, in a large bowl
   combine all the vegetables, herbs, blueberries and avocado.
   Add avocado oil and toss gently to combine. Season well
   with salt and pepper, and top with pumpkin seeds and feta.

4 Serve cutlets on top of salad.

Ⓕ MACROS Cals : **893** CHO : **31g** P : **51g** Fat : **72g**
Ⓜ MACROS Cals : **948** CHO : **31g** P : **59g** Fat : **74g**

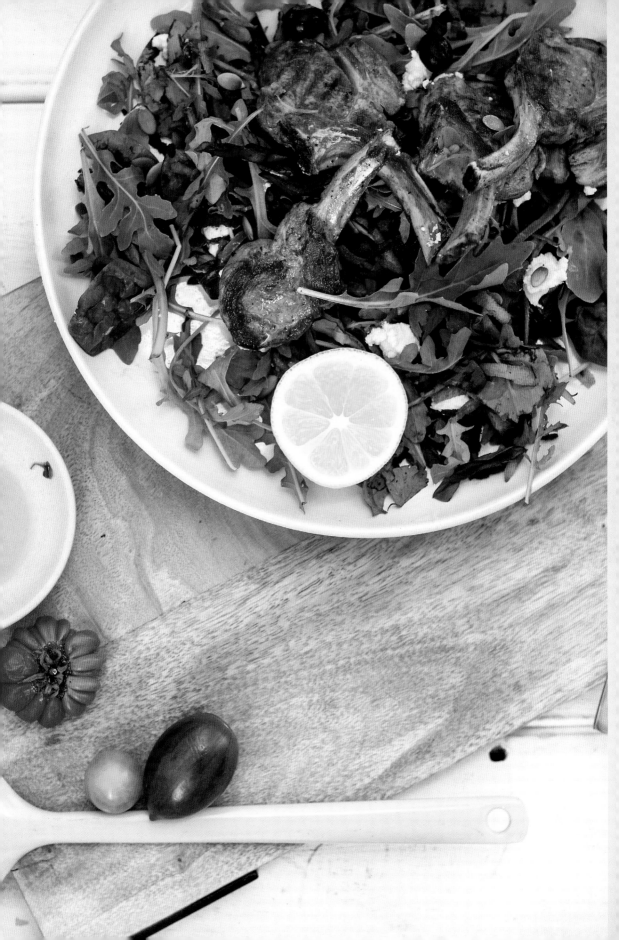

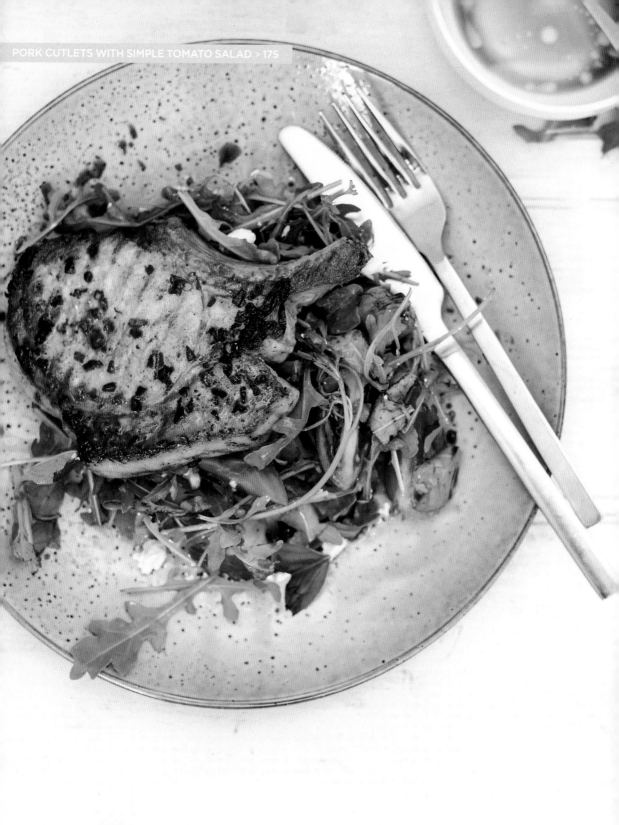

PORK CUTLETS WITH SPINACH & FENNEL SALAD

SERVES Ⓕ Ⓜ 2   PREP : 10 MINUTES + 1–2 HOURS MARINATING   COOK : 10 MINUTES

2 × 120g pork cutlets /
  2 × 150g pork cutlets
1 tablespoon extra-virgin
  olive oil
1 teaspoon sage or chilli flakes
¼ teaspoon sea salt

SPINACH & FENNEL SALAD
100g spinach leaves
1 fennel bulb, thinly sliced
½ avocado, diced
½ cup almonds
sea salt and pepper, to taste

DRESSING
½ avocado
1 tablespoon tahini
1 lemon, juiced
1 tablespoon extra-virgin
  olive oil
¼ teaspoon sea salt

1   Marinate pork cutlets in oil, sage or chilli flakes and sea salt for 1–2 hours.

2   To make the dressing, place all the dressing ingredients plus 1 tablespoon of water in a food processor or blender and blitz until smooth.

3   To make Spinach & Fennel Salad: In a large bowl, place spinach and fennel with 1–2 tablespoons of dressing. Gently massage to combine. Add avocado and almonds, season well with salt and pepper and drizzle with extra dressing if required. Remaining dressing will keep in an airtight glass jar in the fridge for up to 5 days.

4   Drain marinade into a frypan preheated over medium–high heat before adding cutlets and cooking for 6–8 minutes per side, or until cooked to your liking. Rest for 5 minutes. Serve alongside the salad.

Ⓕ MACROS Cals : 962 CHO : 20g P : 43g Fat : 74g
Ⓜ MACROS Cals : 1051 CHO : 20g P : 49g Fat : 79g

PORK CUTLETS WITH SIMPLE TOMATO SALAD

SERVES Ⓕ Ⓜ 2   PREP : 10 MINUTES + 1–2 HOURS MARINATING   COOK : 10 MINUTES

2 × 120g pork cutlets /
  2 × 150g pork cutlets
1 tablespoon extra-virgin
  olive oil
1 teaspoon sage or chilli flakes
¼ teaspoon sea salt

SIMPLE TOMATO SALAD
250g heirloom tomatoes, halved
60g rocket leaves
1 bunch basil, roughly chopped
sea salt and pepper, to taste
1 tablespoon balsamic vinegar
1 tablespoon extra-virgin
  olive oil
100g goat's feta

1   Marinate pork cutlets in oil, sage or chilli flakes and sea salt for 1–2 hours

2   Drain marinade into a frypan preheated over medium–high heat before adding cutlets and cooking for 6–8 minutes per side, or until cooked to your liking. Rest for 5 minutes before serving.

3   To make Simple Tomato Salad: In a large bowl, combine tomatoes, rocket and basil, and season well with salt and pepper. In a small bowl, whisk together balsamic vinegar and olive oil. To serve, crumble feta over the top and drizzle dressing over the salad. Serve pork cutlets onto of the salad.

Ⓕ MACROS Cals : 657 CHO : 10g P : 37g Fat : 45g
Ⓜ MACROS Cals : 746 CHO : 10g P : 43g Fat : 50g

CHICKEN THIGHS WITH BROCCOLI & KALE SALAD

SERVES ⓕ Ⓜ 2   PREP : 10 MINUTES + 1–2 HOURS MARINATING   COOK : 10 MINUTES

240g free-range chicken thigh
fillets / 300g free-range
chicken thigh fillets
¼ cup extra-virgin olive oil
sea salt and pepper, to taste

BROCCOLI & KALE SALAD
1 head of broccoli, cut into
florets
50g kale, finely chopped
½ tablespoon cold-pressed
extra-virgin coconut oil
¼ cup flaked almonds
2 tablespoons goji berries
¼ large avocado, diced
2 tablespoons extra-virgin
olive oil
½ lemon, juiced
¼ teaspoon sea salt
30g goat's feta

1   Marinate chicken in olive oil, sea salt and pepper for
    1–2 hours.

2   Bring a small saucepan of water to the boil. Place broccoli
    in a colander or steamer basket, cover with a lid and lightly
    steam for 4–5 minutes. Remove from the colander or
    steamer basket and set aside in a large bowl to cool.

3   Drain marinade into a frypan preheated over medium heat
    before adding chicken and cooking on both sides for
    10 minutes, or until golden and cooked through. Set aside.

4   Melt coconut oil in a frypan over medium heat, add the kale
    and sauté until soft. Add to the bowl with broccoli. Top with
    almonds, goji berries and avocado.

5   Combine olive oil, lemon juice and salt in a small bowl and
    toss through the salad. Crumble feta on top and serve salad
    alongside the chicken.

ⓕ   MACROS   Cals : 850   CHO : 39g   P : 40g   Fat : 66g
Ⓜ   MACROS   Cals : 893   CHO : 39g   P : 46g   Fat : 69g

GLUTEN-FREE CHICKEN SCHNITZ WITH BUTTERED GREENS

SERVES ⓕ Ⓜ 4   PREP : 10 MINUTES   COOK : 15 MINUTES

1 free-range egg
1 cup almond meal
2 lemons (1 zested, 1 quartered)
sea salt and pepper, to taste
500g free-range chicken breast
fillets, halved / 600g free-
range chicken breast fillets,
halved
2 tablespoons cold-pressed
extra-virgin coconut oil
4 cups chopped broccolini
4 cups diced zucchini
120g grass-fed butter

1   In a small bowl, beat the egg. In a separate bowl, combine
    almond meal and lemon zest, and season well with salt and
    pepper. Lightly coat each chicken piece in the egg, followed
    by the almond mix.

2   Heat oil in a frypan over low to medium heat, add chicken
    and cook for 5 minutes each side, or until lightly golden.

3   To make Buttered Greens: While the chicken is cooking,
    bring a small saucepan of water to the boil. Place broccolini
    and zucchini in a colander or steamer basket, cover with a
    lid and steam for 4–5 minutes. Toss steamed greens with
    butter and season well with salt. Serve the chicken schnitzel
    with lemon quarters alongside greens.

ⓕ   MACROS   Cals : 677   CHO : 17g   P : 40g   Fat : 51g
Ⓜ   MACROS   Cals : 697   CHO : 17g   P : 44g   Fat : 51g

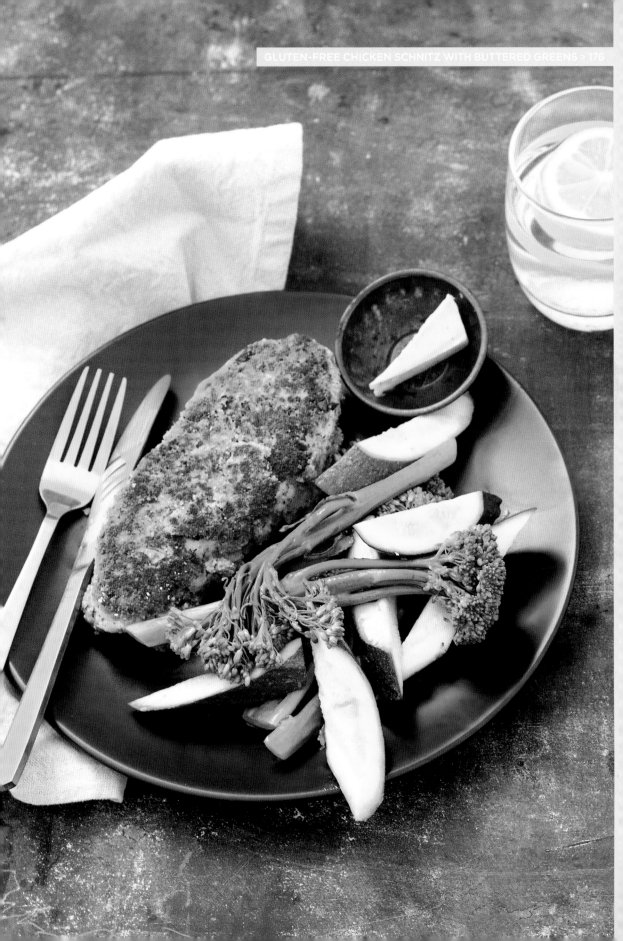

CHICKEN THIGHS WITH SIMPLE GREEK SALAD > 179

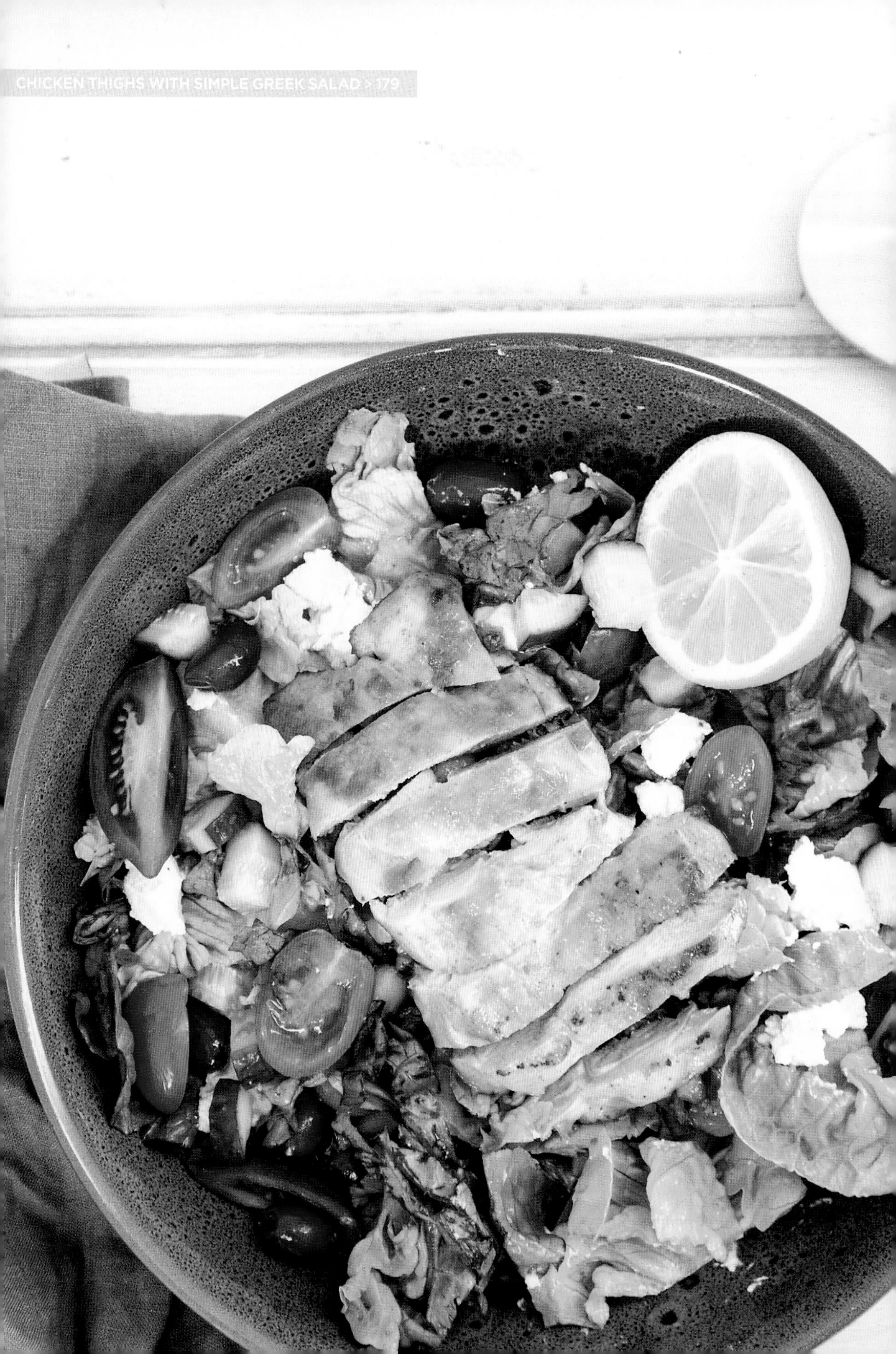

GLUTEN-FREE CHICKEN SCHNITZ WITH SIMPLE TOMATO SALAD

SERVES (F) (M) 4   PREP : 10 MINUTES + 1–2 HOURS MARINATING   COOK : 15 MINUTES

1 free-range egg
1 cup almond meal
2 lemons (1 zested, 1 quartered)
sea salt and pepper, to taste
500g free-range chicken breast
   fillets, halved / 600g free-
   range chicken breast fillets,
   halved
2 tablespoons cold-pressed
   extra-virgin coconut oil
2 tablespoons chopped fresh
   parsley

SIMPLE TOMATO SALAD
500g heirloom tomatoes, halved
120g rocket leaves
1 bunch basil, leaves chopped
sea salt and pepper, to taste
2 tablespoons balsamic vinegar
2 tablespoons extra-virgin
   olive oil
150g goat's feta

1   In a small bowl, beat the egg. In a separate bowl, combine almond meal and lemon zest, and season well with salt and pepper. Lightly coat each chicken piece in the egg, followed by the almond mix.

2   Heat coconut oil in a frypan over low to medium heat, add the chicken and cook for 5 minutes each side, or until lightly golden.

3   To make Tomato Salad: While the chicken is cooking, in a large bowl combine tomatoes, rocket and basil, and season well with salt and pepper. In a small bowl, whisk together balsamic vinegar and olive oil. To serve, crumble feta over the top and drizzle dressing over the salad.

4   Serve chicken schnitzel scattered with parsley, with salad on the side.

(F) MACROS   Cals : **430**   CHO : **11g**   P : **38g**   Fat : **25g**
(M) MACROS   Cals : **459**   CHO : **11g**   P : **43g**   Fat : **25g**

CHICKEN THIGHS WITH SIMPLE GREEK SALAD

SERVES (F) (M) 2   PREP : 10 MINUTES + 1–2 HOURS MARINATING   COOK : 10 MINUTES

240g free-range chicken thigh
   fillets / 300g free-range
   chicken thigh fillets
½ cup extra-virgin olive oil
sea salt and pepper, to taste
½ cos lettuce, leaves torn
100g cherry tomatoes,
   quartered
½ cucumber, diced
15g goats feta, crumbled
10 black olives, halved and
   pitted
1 lemon, juiced

1   Marinate chicken in ¼ cup oil, salt and pepper for 1–2 hours.

2   Drain marinade into a frypan preheated over medium heat before adding chicken and cooking on both sides for 10 minutes, or until golden and cooked through. Rest for 5 minutes before serving.

3   While the chicken is cooking, in a large bowl combine lettuce, cherry tomatoes, cucumber, feta and olives. In a small bowl, whisk together remaining olive oil and lemon juice, and toss through the salad. Season with salt and pepper. Slice the chicken and serve on top of the salad.

(F) MACROS   Cals : **581**   CHO : **6g**   P : **26g**   Fat : **52g**
(M) MACROS   Cals : **624**   CHO : **6g**   P : **32g**   Fat : **55g**

CLEAN CHICKEN PARMA
WITH ZUCCHINI CHIPS

SERVES Ⓕ Ⓜ 4   PREP : 10 MINUTES   COOK : 15 MINUTES

1 free-range egg
1 cup almond or hazelnut meal
1 tablespoon coconut flour
400g free-range chicken thigh
  fillets
½ cup cold-pressed extra-virgin
  coconut oil
4 slices ham, free range
Sugar-free Tomato Sauce
  (see recipe page 205)
2 slices organic hard cheese
sea salt and pepper, to taste

ZUCCHINI CHIPS
1 large zucchini
2 tablespoons cold-pressed
  extra-virgin coconut oil
sea salt, to taste

1 Preheat oven to 180°C and line a baking tray with baking paper.

2 To make Zucchini Chips: Slice zucchini into thin chip-like pieces and toss with oil and salt. Bake for 10–15 minutes.

3 Meanwhile, place egg in a small bowl and whisk well. In a separate bowl, combine almond or hazelnut meal and coconut flour.

4 Cover chicken thighs well in egg, then coat well in the flour mix.

5 Heat coconut oil in a large frypan over medium–high heat and shallow-fry chicken on both sides for 5 minutes, or until lightly browned.

6 Transfer chicken from the frypan onto the lined baking tray. Place ham on top of chicken, add 1–2 tablespoons Sugar-free Tomato Sauce and top with cheese. Bake in the oven for 10 minutes, or until the cheese has melted.

7 Finish the parmas and chips off under the grill until crispy, and serve.

Ⓕ MACROS Cals : **800** CHO : **12g**   P : **41g**   Fat : **59g**
Ⓜ MACROS Cals : **800** CHO : **12g**   P : **41g**   Fat : **59g**

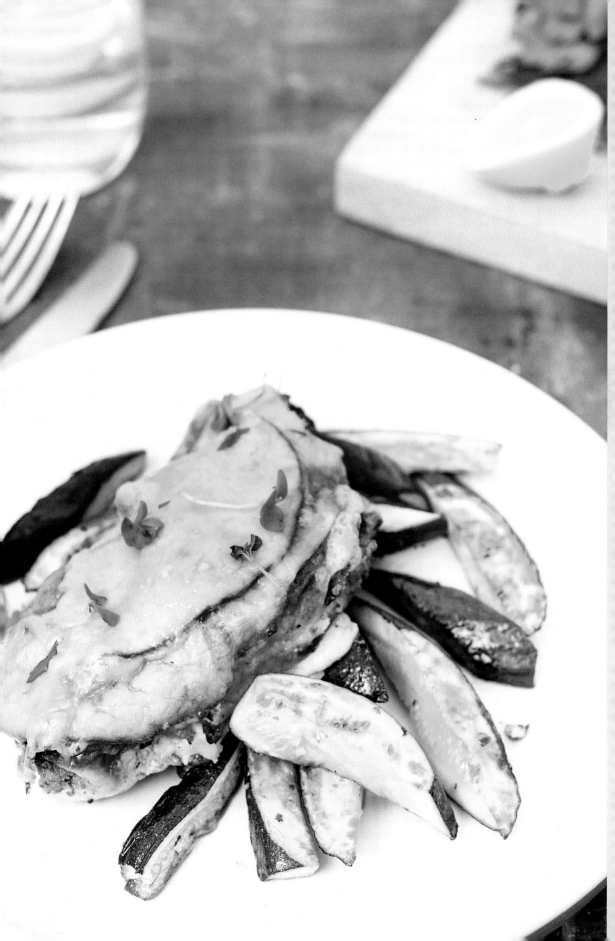

CLEAN CHICKEN PARMA WITH BUTTERED GREENS

SERVES Ⓕ Ⓜ 4   PREP : 15 MINUTES   COOK : 15 MINUTES

1 free-range egg
1 cup almond or hazelnut meal
1 tablespoon coconut flour
400g free-range chicken thigh
    fillets
½ cup cold-pressed extra-virgin
    coconut oil
4 slices ham, free range
Sugar-free Tomato Sauce
    (see recipe page 205)
2 slices organic hard cheese
sea salt and pepper, to taste

BUTTERED GREENS
4 cups roughly chopped
    broccolini
4 cups diced zucchini
120g grass-fed butter
sea salt, to taste

1   Preheat oven to 180°C and line a baking tray with baking paper.

2   Place egg in a small bowl and whisk well. In a separate bowl, combine almond or hazelnut meal and coconut flour.

3   Cover chicken thighs well in egg, then coat well in the flour mix.

4   Heat coconut oil in a large frypan over medium–high heat and shallow-fry chicken on both sides for 5 minutes, or until lightly browned.

5   Transfer the chicken to the lined baking tray. Place ham on top of chicken, add 1–2 tablespoons Sugar-free Tomato Sauce and top with cheese. Bake in the oven for 10 minutes, or until the cheese has melted.

6   To make Buttered Greens: While the chicken parma is baking, bring a small saucepan of water to the boil. Place broccolini and zucchini in a colander or steamer basket, cover with a lid and steam for 4–5 minutes. Toss steamed greens with butter and season well with salt.

7   Serve the schnitzel alongside buttered greens.

Ⓕ MACROS Cals : **907** CHO : **17g** P : **43g** Fat : **69g**
Ⓜ MACROS Cals : **907** CHO : **17g** P : **43g** Fat : **69g**

CLEAN CHICKEN PARMA WITH SUPER SALAD

SERVES (F)(M) 2   PREP : 15 MINUTES   COOK : 15 MINUTES

1 free-range egg
½ cup almond or hazelnut meal
1 tablespoon coconut flour
200g free-range chicken thigh
  fillets
¼ cup cold-pressed extra-virgin
  coconut oil
2 slices ham, free range
Sugar-free Tomato Sauce
  (see recipe page 205)
2 slices organic hard cheese
sea salt and pepper, to taste

SUPER SALAD
60g spinach and rocket leaves
40g red cabbage, finely
  chopped
1 carrot, grated
1 raw beetroot, grated
125g cherry tomatoes, halved
¼ bunch coriander, roughly
  chopped
¼ bunch basil, roughly chopped
100g blueberries
1 avocado, diced
1 tablespoon avocado oil
sea salt and pepper, to taste
¼ cup pumpkin seeds
50g goat's feta

1 Preheat oven to 180°C and line a baking tray with baking paper.

2 Place egg in a small bowl and whisk well. In a separate bowl, combine almond or hazelnut meal and coconut flour.

3 Cover chicken thighs well in egg, then coat well in the flour mix.

4 Heat coconut oil in a large frypan over medium–high heat and shallow-fry chicken on both sides for 5 minutes, or until lightly browned.

5 Transfer the chicken to the lined baking tray. Place ham on top of chicken, add 1–2 tablespoons Sugar-free Tomato Sauce and top with cheese. Bake in the oven for 10 minutes, or until the cheese has melted.

6 To make Super Salad: While the chicken parma is baking, in a large bowl, combine all the vegetables, herbs, blueberries and avocado. Add avocado oil and toss gently to combine. Season well with salt and pepper, and top with pumpkin seeds and feta.

7 Serve the salad alongside the chicken.

(F) MACROS Cals : 1132 CHO : 38g P : 64g Fat : 81g
(M) MACROS Cals : 1132 CHO : 38g P : 64g Fat : 81g

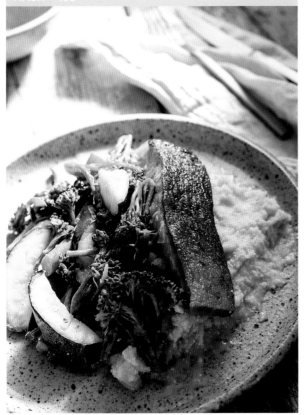
SALMON WITH BUTTERED GREENS & CAULIFLOWER MASH > 185

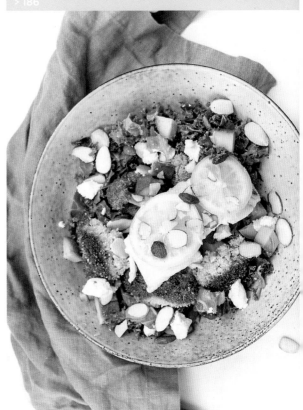
OVEN-BAKED FISH WITH BROCCOLI & KALE SALAD > 186

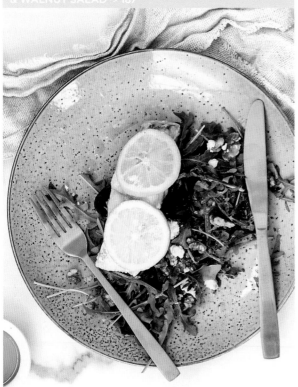
OVEN-BAKED FISH WITH BEETROOT, GOAT'S FETA & WALNUT SALAD > 187

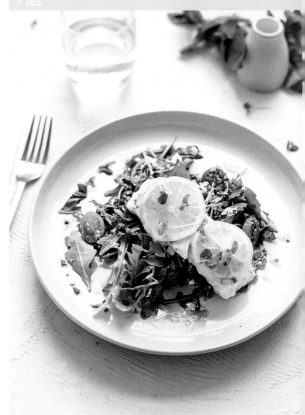
OVEN-BAKED FISH WITH SIMPLE TOMATO SALAD > 185

SALMON WITH BUTTERED GREENS & CAULIFLOWER MASH

SERVES Ⓕ Ⓜ 2   PREP : 10 MINUTES   COOK : 20 MINUTES

2 × 120g salmon fillets,
  preferably wild caught /
  2 × 150g salmon fillets,
  preferably wild caught
sea salt, to taste

BUTTERED GREENS
2 cups roughly chopped
  broccolini
2 cups diced zucchini
60g grass-fed butter
sea salt, to taste

CAULIFLOWER MASH
1 medium head of cauliflower,
  cut into florets
2 tablespoons grass-fed butter
sea salt, to taste

1   Preheat oven to 180°C. Line two large pieces of foil with a square of baking paper. Place the salmon on the baking paper and season well. Wrap the salmon to form a parcel, sealing the edges by folding over the foil, and place on a baking tray. Bake for 20 minutes, or until cooked to your liking.

2   To make Buttered Greens: While the salmon is cooking, bring a small saucepan of water to the boil. Place broccolini and zucchini in a colander or steamer basket, cover with a lid and steam for 4–5 minutes. Remove from the colander or steamer basket and set aside to cool. Toss steamed greens with butter and season well with salt.

3   To make Cauliflower Mash: Place cauliflower in the colander or steamer basket and steam for 5 minutes, or until soft. Mash cauliflower with butter and season with salt to taste.

4   Serve the salmon on top of the greens and mash.

Ⓕ   MACROS   Cals : **701**   CHO : **32g**   P : **38g**   Fat : **49g**
Ⓜ   MACROS   Cals : **759**   CHO : **32g**   P : **45g**   Fat : **53g**

OVEN-BAKED FISH WITH SIMPLE TOMATO SALAD

SERVES Ⓕ Ⓜ 2   PREP : 10 MINUTES   COOK : 15 MINUTES

2 × 120g fillets of firm white fish,
  such as barramundi / 2 × 175g
  fillets of firm white fish, such
  as barramundi
2 tablespoons extra-virgin
  olive oil
sea salt and pepper, to taste
1 lemon, sliced

SIMPLE TOMATO SALAD
250g heirloom tomatoes, halved
60g rocket leaves
1 bunch chopped basil leaves
1 tablespoon balsamic vinegar
1 tablespoon extra-virgin olive oil
100g goat's feta

1   Preheat oven to 200°C. Line two large pieces of foil with a square of baking paper. Place the fish, skin side down, on the baking paper. Drizzle with olive oil and season well. Place slices of lemon on top of each piece of fish. Wrap the fish in foil to form a parcel, sealing the edges by folding over the foil, and place on a baking tray. Bake for 10–15 minutes. Check the fish and if not cooked to your liking, re-seal and return to the oven for a few extra minutes.

2   To make Simple Tomato Salad: While the fish is cooking, in a large bowl combine tomatoes, rocket and basil, and season well. In a small bowl, whisk together the balsamic vinegar and olive oil. To serve, crumble feta over the top, drizzle dressing over the salad and top with the fish.

Ⓕ   MACROS   Cals : **465**   CHO : **10g**   P : **36g**   Fat : **33g**
Ⓜ   MACROS   Cals : **516**   CHO : **10g**   P : **47g**   Fat : **33g**

OVEN-BAKED FISH WITH BROCCOLI & KALE SALAD

SERVES Ⓕ Ⓜ 2   PREP : 5 MINUTES   COOK : 15 MINUTES

2 × 120g fillets of firm white
fish, such as barramundi /
2 × 175g fillets of firm white
fish, such as barramundi
2 tablespoons extra-virgin
olive oil
sea salt and pepper, to taste
1 lemon, sliced

BROCCOLI & KALE SALAD
1 head of broccoli, cut into
florets
50g kale, finely sliced
½ tablespoon cold-pressed
extra-virgin coconut oil
¼ cup flaked almonds
2 tablespoons goji berries
¼ large avocado, diced
2 tablespoons extra-virgin
olive oil
½ lemon, juiced
¼ teaspoon sea salt
30g goat's feta

1   Preheat oven to 200°C.

2   Take two pieces of foil, large enough to wrap each fish fillet, and line each piece with a square of baking paper.

3   Place the fish, skin side down, on the baking paper. Drizzle with olive oil and season well with salt and pepper. Place 2–4 slices of lemon on top of each piece of fish. Wrap the fish in foil to form a parcel, sealing the edges by folding over the foil, and place on a baking tray. Bake for 10–15 minutes. Check the fish and if not cooked to your liking, simply re-seal the foil and place back in the oven for a few extra minutes

4   To make Broccoli & Kale Salad: Bring a small saucepan of water to the boil. Place broccoli in a colander or steamer basket, cover with a lid and steam for 4–5 minutes. Remove from the colander or steamer basket and set aside in a large bowl to cool.

5   Melt coconut oil in a frypan over medium heat, add the kale and sauté until soft. Add to the bowl containing the broccoli. Top with almonds, goji berries and avocado.

6   Combine olive oil, lemon juice and salt in a small bowl and toss through the salad. Crumble feta on top.

7   Serve the salad alongside the fish.

Ⓕ   MACROS   Cals : **663**   CHO : **39g**   P : **40g**   Fat : **45g**
Ⓜ   MACROS   Cals : **714**   CHO : **39g**   P : **51g**   Fat : **45g**

OVEN-BAKED FISH WITH BEETROOT, GOAT'S FETA & WALNUT SALAD

SERVES Ⓕ Ⓜ 2   PREP : 10 MINUTES   COOK : 45 MINUTES

2 × 120g fillets of firm white
  fish, such as barramundi /
  2 × 175g fillets of firm white
  fish, such as bararmundi
2 tablespoons extra-virgin
  olive oil
sea salt and pepper, to taste
1 lemon, sliced

**BEETROOT, GOAT'S FETA
& WALNUT SALAD**
2 large beetroots (about tennis
  ball size each)
2 tablespoons cold-pressed
  extra-virgin coconut oil
¼ cup walnuts
1 tablespoon organic rice malt
  syrup
100g rocket leaves
40g goat's feta, crumbled

DRESSING
¼ cup extra-virgin olive oil
1 tablespoon apple cider
  vinegar
½ teaspoon sea salt

1 Preheat oven to 180°C and line a baking tray with baking
   paper.

2 Prick beetroot with a fork all over, toss through coconut oil
   and place on the baking tray. Bake for 45 minutes, or until
   tender. Set aside to cool. Peel and dice.

3 About halfway through baking the beetroot, prepare the
   fish. Take two pieces of foil, large enough to wrap each fish
   fillet, and line each piece with a square of baking paper.

4 Place the fish, skin side down, on the baking paper. Drizzle
   with olive oil and season well with salt and pepper. Place
   2–4 slices of lemon on top of each piece of fish. Wrap the
   fish in foil to form a parcel, sealing the edges by folding over
   the foil, and place on a baking tray. Bake for 10–15 minutes.
   Check the fish and if not cooked to your liking, simply re-seal
   the foil and place back in the oven for a few extra minutes.

5 Heat a frypan over low heat, add walnuts and rice malt
   syrup, and sauté lightly. Set aside to cool.

6 Place dressing ingredients in a small bowl and whisk to
   combine.

7 Place rocket and beetroot in a large bowl and toss through
   the dressing. Scatter feta and walnuts on top.

8 Serve the salad alongside the fish.

Ⓕ MACROS Cals : **660** CHO : **16g** P : **30g** Fat : **56g**
Ⓜ MACROS Cals : **711** CHO : **16g** P : **41g** Fat : **56g**

GREEN VEGIE SLICE WITH SIMPLE GREEK SALAD

SERVES (F) (M) 4 / 3   PREP : 10 MINUTES   COOK : 30 MINUTES

¼ cup cold-pressed extra-virgin coconut oil
1 zucchini, finely chopped
½ bunch broccolini, finely chopped
5 free-range eggs
1 cup almond or macadamia nut flour
sea salt and pepper, to taste

SIMPLE GREEK SALAD

½ cos lettuce, leaves roughly chopped / 1 cos lettuce, leaves roughly chopped
100g cherry tomatoes, quartered / 200g cherry tomatoes, quartered
½ cucumber, diced / 1 cucumber, diced
15g goat's feta / 30g goat's feta
10 black olives, halved and pitted / 20 black olives, halved and pitted
2 tablespoons extra-virgin olive oil / ¼ cup extra-virgin olive oil
1 lemon, juiced
sea salt and pepper, to taste

1   Preheat oven to 180°C. Grease a quiche tin or baking pan with 1 teaspoon of the coconut oil.

2   Place the zucchini and broccoli in a large bowl.

3   Whisk eggs in a separate bowl then add to vegies, along with the remaining oil and the flour. Stir well and season with salt and pepper to taste.

4   Pour into the quiche tin or pan and bake for 20–30 minutes, or until cooked through. Allow to cool, then slice into 6 serves.

5   To make the Greek Salad: While the slice is cooking, in a large bowl combine lettuce, cherry tomatoes, cucumber, feta and olives. In a small bowl, whisk together olive oil and lemon juice and toss through the salad. Season well with salt and pepper.

6   Serve the Greek Salad alongside the slice. Remaining slice will keep in the fridge for 4–5 days.

(F) MACROS   Cals : **569**   CHO : **11g**   P : **11g**   Fat : **55g**
(M) MACROS   Cals : **767**   CHO : **13g**   P : **17g**   Fat : **75g**

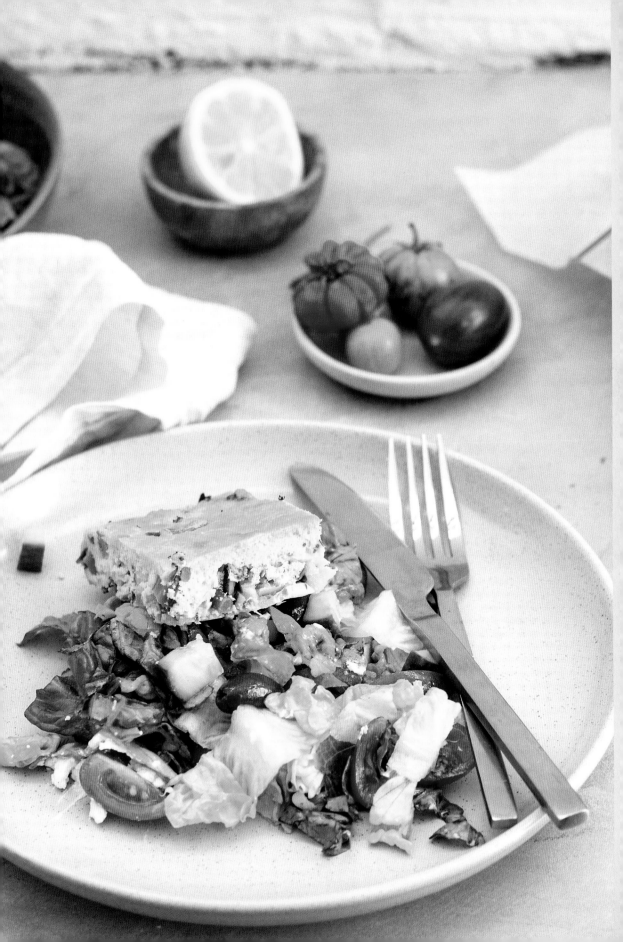

SALMON WITH SIMPLE GREEK SALAD

SERVES Ⓕ Ⓜ 2   PREP : 10 MINUTES   COOK : 20 MINUTES

2 × 120g salmon fillets,
    preferably wild caught /
    2 × 150g salmon fillets,
    preferably wild caught
sea salt, to taste

SIMPLE GREEK SALAD
½ cos lettuce, leaves roughly
    chopped
125g cherry tomatoes, quartered
½ cucumber, diced
15g goat's feta / 30g goat's feta
10 black olives, halved and pitted
2 tablespoons extra-virgin
    olive oil
1 lemon, juiced
sea salt and pepper, to taste

1   Preheat oven to 180°C.

2   Take two pieces of foil, large enough to wrap each salmon
    fillet, and line each piece with a square of baking paper.
    Place the salmon on the baking paper and season well with
    salt. Wrap the salmon in foil to form a parcel, sealing the
    edges by folding over the foil, and place on a baking tray.
    Bake for 20 minutes, or until cooked to your liking.

3   To make Greek Salad: While the salmon is cooking, in a
    large bowl combine lettuce, cherry tomatoes, cucumber,
    feta and olives. In a small bowl, whisk together olive oil and
    lemon juice, and toss through the salad. Season well with
    salt and pepper.

4   Serve the salad alongside the salmon fillet.

Ⓕ   MACROS   Cals : **416**   CHO : **4g**   P : **26g**   Fat : **33g**
Ⓜ   MACROS   Cals : **500**   CHO : **4g**   P : **34g**   Fat : **38g**

GREEN VEGIE SLICE WITH SPINACH & FENNEL SALAD

SERVES Ⓕ Ⓜ 4 / 3   PREP : 10 MINUTES   COOK : 30 MINUTES

¼ cup cold-pressed extra-virgin coconut oil
1 zucchini, finely sliced
½ bunch broccolini, finely chopped
5 free-range eggs
1 cup almond or macadamia flour
sea salt and pepper, to taste

SPINACH & FENNEL SALAD
100g spinach leaves
1 fennel bulb, thinly sliced
½ avocado, diced
½ cup almonds
sea salt and pepper, to taste

DRESSING
½ avocado
1 tablespoon tahini
1 lemon, juiced
1 tablespoon extra-virgin olive oil
¼ teaspoon sea salt

1 Preheat oven to 180°C. Grease a quiche tin or baking pan with 1 teaspoon of the coconut oil.

2 Place the zucchini and broccolini in a large bowl.

3 Whisk eggs in a separate bowl then add to vegies, along with the remaining oil and the flour. Stir well and season with salt and pepper to taste.

4 Pour into the quiche tin or pan and bake for 20–30 minutes, or until cooked through. Allow to cool, then slice into 6 serves.

5 While the slice is cooking, make the dressing: Place all the dressing ingredients plus 1 tablespoon of water in a food processor or blender and blitz until smooth.

6 To make Spinach & Fennel Salad: In a large bowl, place spinach and fennel with 1–2 tablespoons of dressing. Gently massage to combine. Add avocado and almonds, season well with salt and pepper and drizzle with extra dressing, if required. Remaining dressing will keep in the fridge for up to 5 days.

7 Serve the salad alongside the slice. Remaining slice will keep in the fridge for 4–5 days.

Ⓕ MACROS Cals : **484** CHO : **16g** P : **16g** Fat : **42g**
Ⓜ MACROS Cals : **645** CHO : **21g** P : **22g** Fat : **56g**

SIDES

All of your favourite LCHF sides in one place means that you can start to create your own meals each week. All you need to do is pair a side dish with your choice of protein and you have everything you need for a well-balanced plate that is so simple and tasty.

BUTTERED GREENS

SERVES (F) (M) 4   PREP : 5 MINUTES   COOK : 10 MINUTES

4 cups chopped broccolini
4 cups diced zucchini
120g grass-fed butter
sea salt, to taste

1 Bring a small saucepan of water to the boil. Place broccolini and zucchini in a colander or steamer basket, cover with a lid and steam for 4–5 minutes.

2 Toss steamed greens with butter and season with salt.

MACROS   Cals : **263**   CHO : **10g**   P : **4g**   Fat : **24g**

ZUCCHINI CHIPS

SERVES (F) (M) 2   PREP : 5 MINUTES   COOK : 15 MINUTES

1 large zucchini
2 tablespoons cold-pressed
   extra-virgin coconut oil
sea salt, to taste

1 Preheat oven to 180°C and line a baking tray with baking paper.

2 Slice zucchini into thin chip-like pieces and toss with oil and salt. Bake for 10–15 minutes.

3 Finish off under the grill until crispy.

MACROS   Cals : **156**   CHO : **5g**   P : **2g**   Fat : **14g**

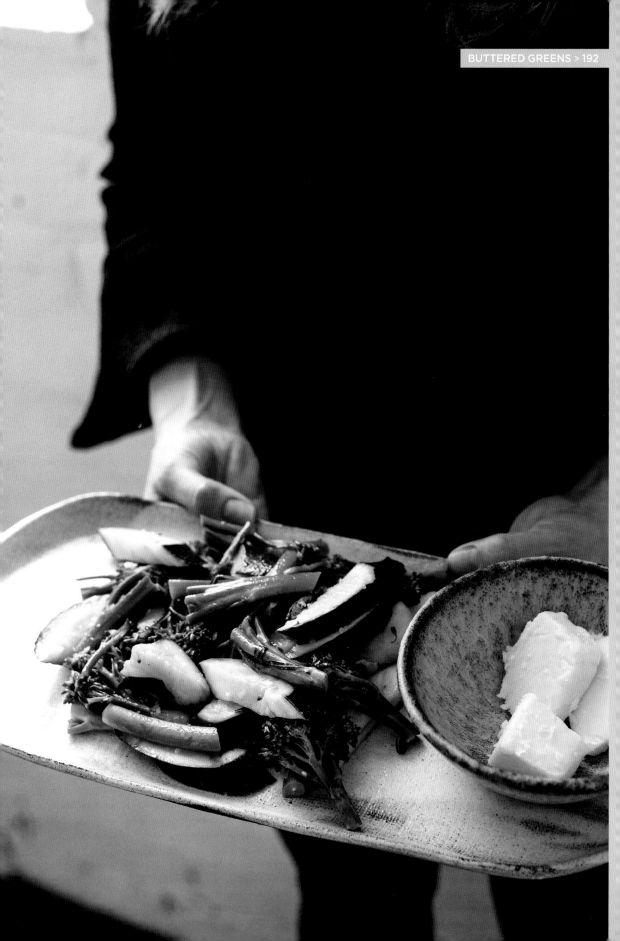

ZUCCHINI CHIPS > 192

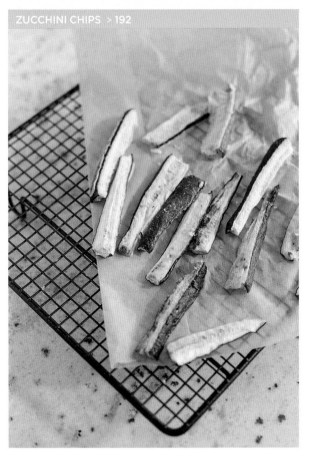

STEAMED BROCCOLINI WITH FETA > 195

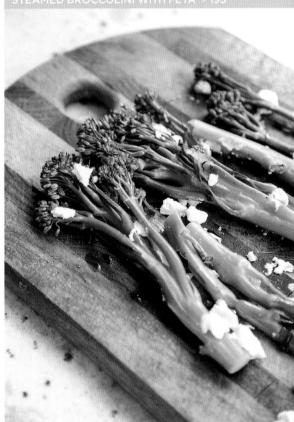

CAULIFLOWER MASH > 195

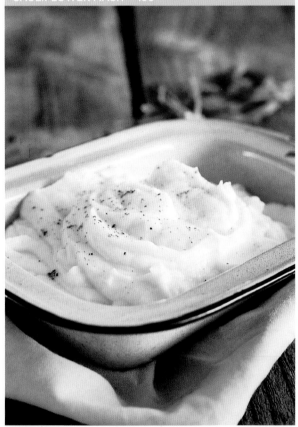

CAULIFLOWER RICE > 195

STEAMED BROCCOLINI WITH FETA

SERVES (F)(M) 1   PREP : 5 MINUTES   COOK : 5 MINUTES

½ bunch broccolini
30g goat's feta
1 tablespoon apple cider
   vinegar
2 tablespoons extra-virgin
   olive oil

1 Bring a small saucepan of water to the boil. Place broccolini
   in a colander or steamer basket, cover with a lid and steam
   for 4–5 minutes. Remove from the colander or steamer
   basket.

2 Crumble feta on top and drizzle with vinegar and oil.

MACROS   Cals : 340 CHO : 4g   P : 8g   Fat : 34g

CAULIFLOWER MASH

SERVES (F)(M) 2   PREP : 5 MINUTES   COOK : 10 MINUTES

1 medium head of cauliflower,
   cut into florets
2 tablespoons grass-fed butter
sea salt, to taste

1 Bring a small saucepan of water to the boil. Place cauliflower
   in a colander or steamer basket, cover with a lid and steam
   for 4–5 minutes. Remove from the colander or steamer
   basket and return to drained saucepan.

2 Mash with the butter and season with salt to taste.

MACROS   Cals : 205 CHO : 22g   P : 8g   Fat : 11g

CAULIFLOWER RICE

SERVES (F)(M) 2   PREP : 5 MINUTES   COOK : 5 MINUTES

1 medium head of cauliflower
2 tablespoons cold-pressed
   extra-virgin coconut oil
sea salt, to taste

1 Thoroughly wash and drain cauliflower. Remove stem, dice
   into small pieces and blitz in a food processor or blender
   until it resembles rice.

2 Heat oil in a large frypan over medium heat and lightly sauté
   cauliflower rice for 5 minutes. Season well with salt.

MACROS   Cals : 90 CHO : 7g   P : 3g   Fat : 7g

SUPER-EASY SIDE SALAD

SERVES (F) (M) 2   PREP : 10 MINUTES

100g rocket leaves
125g cherry tomatoes, halved
1 avocado, diced
2 tablespoons fermented
  vegetables
2 tablespoons extra-virgin
  olive oil
½ lemon, juiced
sea salt and pepper, to taste

1 In a large bowl, combine rocket, cherry tomatoes, avocado
   and fermented vegetables.

2 In a small bowl, whisk together olive oil and lemon juice and
   toss through salad. Season to taste with salt and pepper.

MACROS   Cals : **270**   CHO : **12g**   P : **4g**   Fat : **25g**

SIMPLE GREEK SALAD

SERVES (F) (M) 4   PREP : 10 MINUTES

1 cos lettuce, leaves roughly torn
200g cherry tomatoes, quartered
1 cucumber, diced
30g goat's feta, crumbled
20 black olives, halved and
  pitted
¼ cup extra-virgin olive oil
1 lemon, juiced
sea salt and pepper, to taste

1 In a large bowl, combine lettuce, cherry tomatoes,
   cucumber, feta and olives.

2 In a small bowl, whisk together olive oil and lemon juice and
   toss through salad. Season well with salt and pepper.

MACROS   Cals : **172**   CHO : **6g**   P : **3g**   Fat : **16g**

BROCCOLI & KALE SALAD

SERVES (F) (M) 4   PREP : 10 MINUTES   COOK : 10 MINUTES

2 heads of broccoli, cut into
  florets
100g finely sliced kale
1 tablespoon cold-pressed
  extra-virgin coconut oil
½ cup flaked almonds
¼ cup goji berries
½ large avocado, diced
¼ cup extra-virgin olive oil
½ lemon, juiced
¼ teaspoon sea salt
30g goat's feta

1 Bring a small saucepan of water to the boil. Place broccoli in
   a colander or steamer basket, cover with a lid and steam for
   4–5 minutes. Remove from the colander or steamer basket
   and set aside in a large bowl to cool.

2 Heat coconut oil in a frypan over medium heat, add kale and
   sauté until soft. Add to the bowl with broccoli.

3 Top with almonds, goji berries and avocado.

4 Combine olive oil, lemon juice and salt in a small bowl and
   toss through the salad. Crumble feta on top.

MACROS   Cals : **441**   CHO : **39g**   P : **17g**   Fat : **30g**

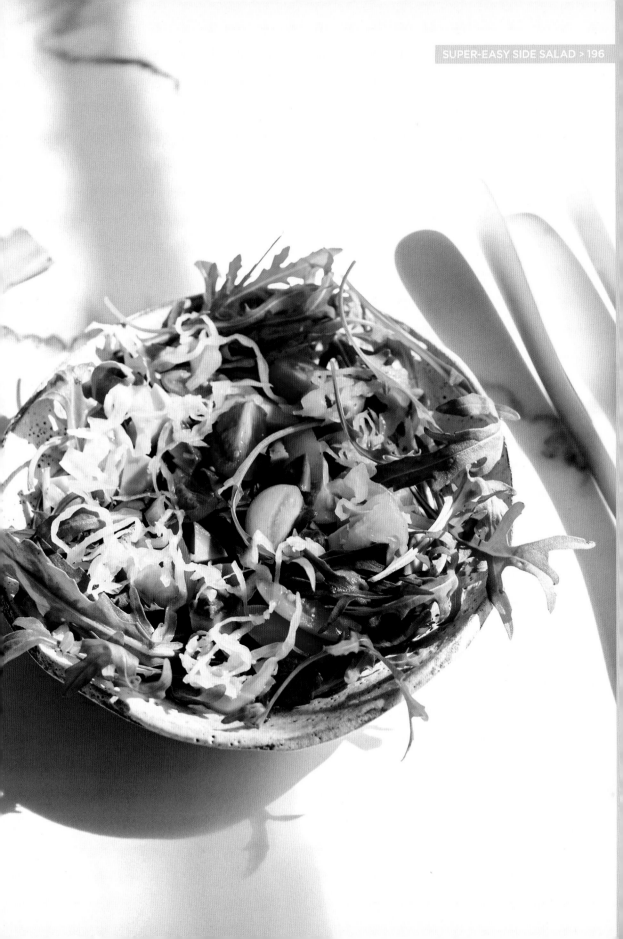

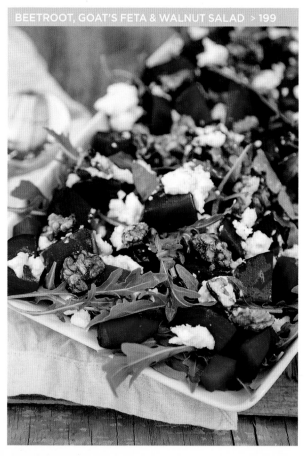

SIMPLE GREEK SALAD > 196

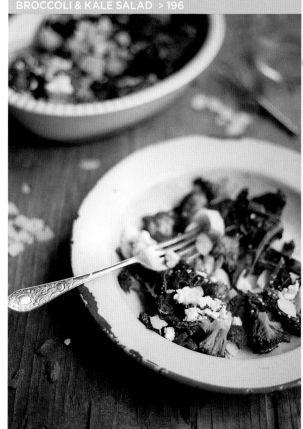

BROCCOLI & KALE SALAD > 196

BEETROOT, GOAT'S FETA & WALNUT SALAD > 199

SUPER SALAD > 199

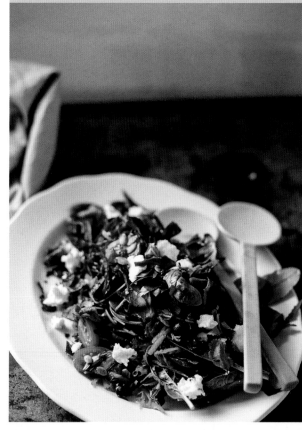

BEETROOT, GOAT'S FETA & WALNUT SALAD

SERVES (F) (M) 4   PREP : 10 MINUTES   COOK : 45 MINUTES

4 large beetroots (about tennis ball size each)
¼ cup cold-pressed extra-virgin coconut oil
½ cup walnuts
2 tablespoons organic rice malt syrup
200g rocket leaves
80g goat's feta, crumbled

DRESSING
¼ cup extra-virgin olive oil
1 tablespoon apple cider vinegar
½ teaspoon sea salt

1 Preheat oven to 180°C and line a baking tray with baking paper.

2 Prick beetroot with a fork all over, toss through coconut oil and place on the baking tray. Bake for 45 minutes, or until tender. Set aside to cool. Peel and dice.

3 Heat a frypan over low heat, add walnuts and rice malt syrup, and sauté lightly. Set aside to cool.

4 Place olive oil, vinegar and salt in a small bowl and whisk to combine.

5 Place rocket and beetroot in a large bowl and toss through the dressing. Scatter feta and walnuts on top.

MACROS   Cals : **438**   CHO : **16g**   P : **7g**   Fat : **41g**

SUPER SALAD

SERVES (F) (M) 2   PREP : 10 MINUTES

60g spinach and rocket leaves
40g finely chopped red cabbage
1 carrot, grated
1 raw beetroot, grated
125g cherry tomatoes, halved
¼ bunch coriander, roughly chopped
¼ bunch basil, roughly chopped
100g blueberries
1 avocado, diced
1 tablespoon avocado oil
sea salt and pepper, to taste
¼ cup pumpkin seeds
50g goat's feta, crumbled

1 In a large bowl, combine all the vegetables, herbs, blueberries and avocado. Add avocado oil and toss gently to combine.

2 Season well with salt and pepper, and top with pumpkin seeds and feta.

MACROS   Cals : **488**   CHO : **31g**   P : **25g**   Fat : **36g**

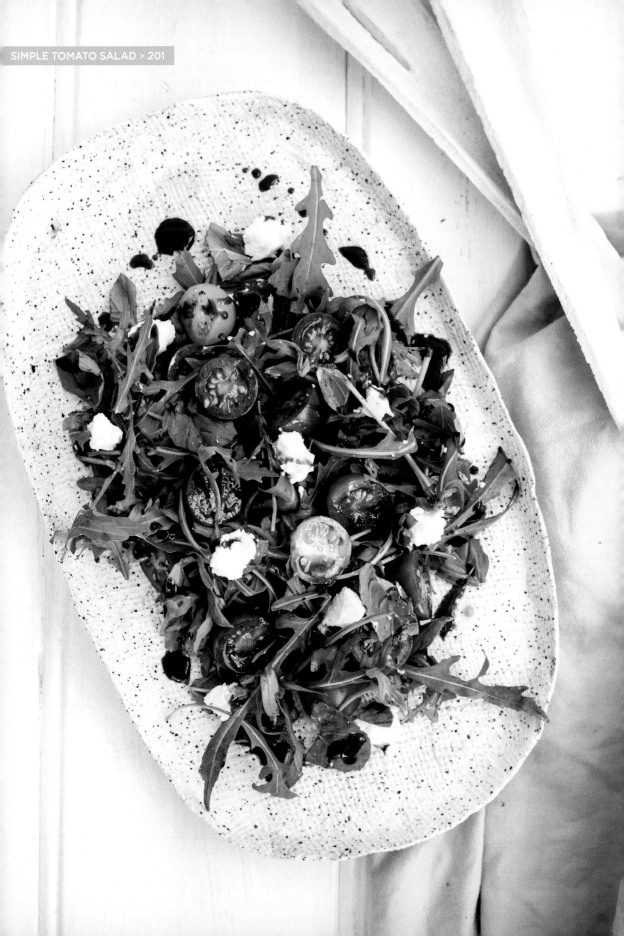

SIMPLE TOMATO SALAD

SERVES (F) (M) 2   PREP : 10 MINUTES

250g heirloom tomatoes, halved
60g rocket leaves
1 bunch basil, roughly chopped
sea salt and pepper, to taste
1 tablespoon balsamic vinegar
1 tablespoon extra-virgin
   olive oil
100g goat's feta

1 In a large bowl, combine tomatoes, rocket and basil, and
   season well with salt and pepper.

2 In a small bowl, whisk together balsamic vinegar and
   olive oil.

3 To serve, crumble feta over the top and drizzle dressing
   over the salad.

MACROS   Cals : **243**   CHO : **10g**   P : **13g**   Fat : **18g**

SPINACH & FENNEL SALAD

SERVES (F) (M) 2   PREP : 10 MINUTES

100g spinach leaves
1 fennel bulb, thinly sliced
½ avocado, diced
½ cup almonds
sea salt and pepper, to taste

DRESSING
½ avocado
1 tablespoon tahini
1 lemon, juiced
1 tablespoon extra-virgin
   olive oil
¼ teaspoon sea salt

1 To make the dressing, place all the dressing ingredients
   plus 1 tablespoon of water in a food processor or blender
   and blitz until smooth.

2 In a large bowl, place spinach and fennel with 1–2
   tablespoons of dressing. Gently massage to combine.

3 Add avocado and almonds, season well with salt and
   pepper and drizzle with extra dressing, if required.
   Remaining dressing will keep in the fridge for up to 5 days.

MACROS   Cals : **548**   CHO : **20g**   P : **19g**   Fat : **47g**

Here are some of my favourite dressings and condiments. You never need to get stuck with the poor-quality ingredients found in nearly every store-bought option. Use the dressings to add variety to your salads and vegetables, and pair the condiments with your favourite main dishes.

PALEO MAYO

MAKES : 1–2 CUPS   PREP : 10 MINUTES

1 free-range egg
1 tablespoon lemon juice
1 tablespoon apple cider vinegar
1 teaspoon Dijon mustard
¾ cup macadamia oil
¼ teaspoon sea salt

1 In a blender or food processor, blend egg, lemon juice, vinegar and mustard.

2 Slowly add oil, 1 tablespoon at a time, continuing to blend.

3 Add salt once a creamy mayonnaise has formed.

4 Transfer to an airtight glass jar and store up until the use-by date on your carton of eggs.

MACROS   Cals : 194   CHO : 0g   P : 2g   Fat : 17g

ALMOND BUTTER DRESSING

SERVES Ⓕ Ⓜ 1–2   PREP : 2 MINUTES

2 tablespoons extra-virgin olive oil
1 tablespoon almond butter
1 lemon, zested and juiced

Place all the ingredients plus 1 tablespoon of water in a small bowl and whisk until well combined. Whisk in a little extra water if a runnier dressing is desired.

MACROS   Cals : 89   CHO : 2g   P : 1g   Fat : 9g

TAHINI DRESSING

SERVES Ⓕ Ⓜ 1–2   PREP : 2 MINUTES

¼ cup tahini
1 lemon, zested and juiced
½ teaspoon garlic powder
½ teaspoon sea salt

Place all the ingredients plus 1 tablespoon of water in a glass jar and whisk well to combine. Whisk in a little extra water if a runnier dressing is desired.

MACROS   Cals : 173   CHO : 4g   P : 6g   Fat : 15g

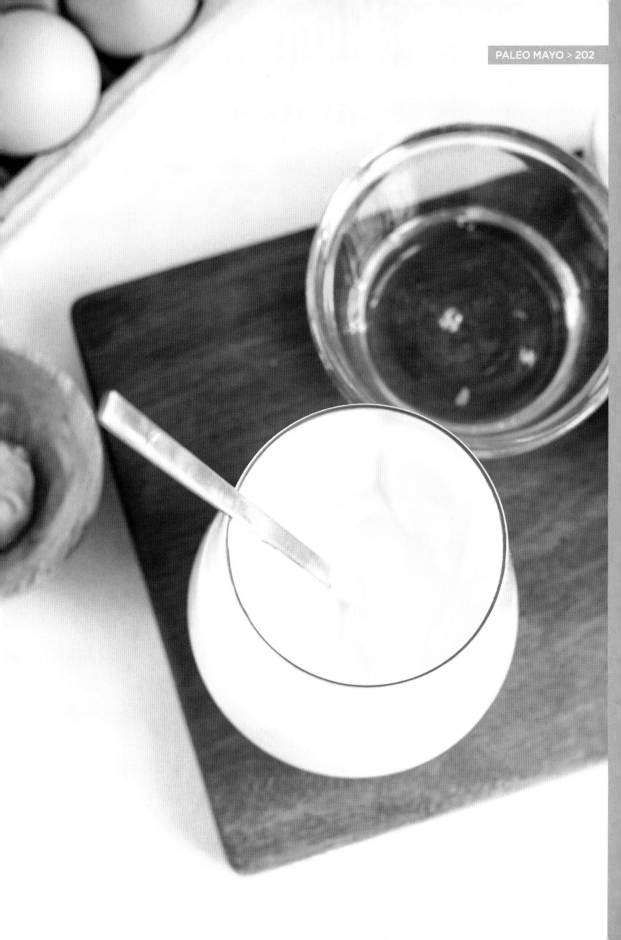

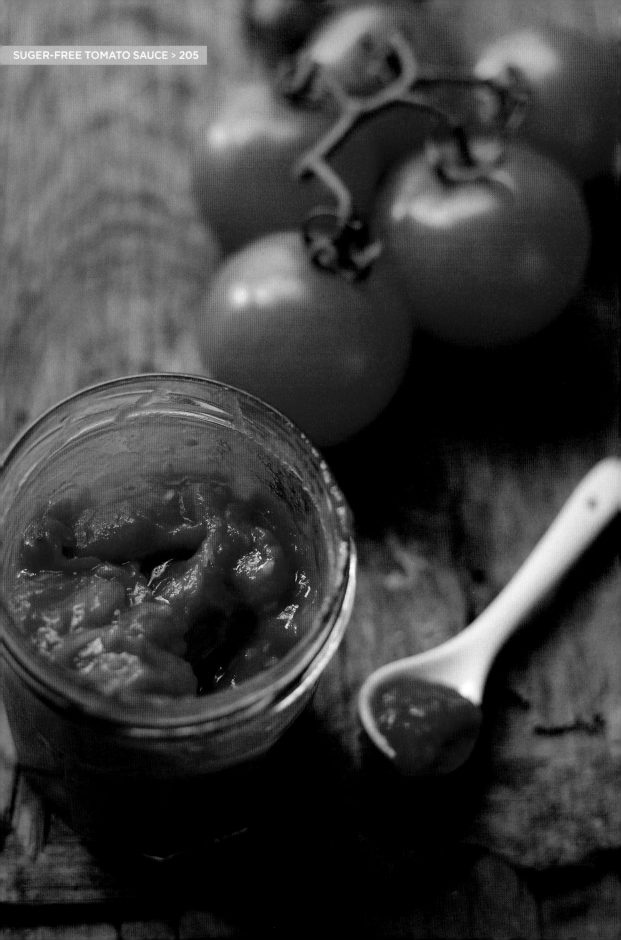

DIJON MUSTARD DRESSING

SERVES (F) (M) 1–2   PREP : 2 MINUTES

1 tablespoon Dijon mustard
1 tablespoon extra-virgin
  olive oil
½ lemon, juiced
¼ teaspoon salt

Place all the ingredients in a small bowl and whisk to combine.

MACROS   Cals : 31   CHO : 0g   P : 0g   Fat : 4g

AVOCADO DRESSING

SERVES (F) (M) 1–2   PREP : 2 MINUTES

½ avocado
⅓ cup extra-virgin olive oil
1 lime, juiced
½ teaspoon garlic powder
½ bunch basil
sea salt and pepper, to taste

Place all the ingredients in a blender or food processor and blitz until smooth and creamy. Blend in a little water if you would like a thinner dressing.

MACROS   Cals : 190   CHO : 2g   P : 0g   Fat : 21g

AVOCADO & TAHINI DRESSING

SERVES (F) (M) 1–2   PREP : 2 MINUTES

½ avocado
1 tablespoon tahini
1 lemon, juiced
1 tablespoon extra-virgin
  olive oil
¼ teaspoon sea salt

Place all the ingredients plus 1 tablespoon of water in a blender or food processor and blitz until smooth.

MACROS   Cals : 94   CHO : 3g   P : 2g   Fat : 9g

SUGAR-FREE TOMATO SAUCE

MAKES : 2–3 CUPS   PREP : 5 MINUTES   COOK : 15 MINUTES

1 teaspoon cold-pressed
  extra-virgin coconut oil
1 garlic clove, crushed
400g can chopped tomatoes
2 tablespoons tomato paste
  (salt reduced)
½ cup apple cider vinegar
¼ teaspoon sea salt
1 tablespoon organic rice
  malt syrup

1   Melt coconut oil in a large saucepan over medium heat, add garlic and cook until brown.

2   Add all remaining ingredients and bring to the boil.

3   Reduce heat and simmer until thick, about 10–15 minutes.

4   Remove from heat and allow to cool. Store in the fridge in an airtight glass container for up to 3 weeks.

MACROS   Cals : 11   CHO : 2g   P : 0g   Fat : 0g

BREADS & MUFFINS

With a focus on nutrient density via LCHF ingredients, you can still get your bread or muffin fix. As your tastebuds evolve and metabolism improves, you'll no longer crave the refined store-bought options.

ALMOST PALEO VEGIE BREAD

MAKES : 10 SLICES   PREP : 10 MINUTES   COOK : 30 MINUTES

2 cups almond meal
½ cup buckwheat flour
1 tablespoon psyllium husks
¼ teaspoon sea salt
1 teaspoon gluten-free baking powder
1 cup grated pumpkin
1 cup grated zucchini
4 free-range eggs, whisked
¼ cup cold-pressed extra-virgin coconut oil, melted
1 tablespoon organic rice malt syrup
1 tablespoon apple cider vinegar

1   Preheat oven to 180°C and line a bread tin with baking paper.
2   In a large bowl, place almond meal, buckwheat flour, psyllium husks, salt and baking powder, and stir to combine.
3   To the bowl add the grated vegetables, eggs, coconut oil, rice malt syrup and vinegar, and mix thoroughly.
4   Scoop into the prepared tin and bake for 30 minutes, or until a skewer inserted into the centre comes out clean.
5   Cool in the tin, cut into 10 slices and store in an airtight container in the fridge for up to 10 days. This bread also freezes well.

MACROS   Cals : 216   CHO : 11g   P : 9g   Fat : 16g

SAVOURY ZUCCHINI BREAD

MAKES : 12 SLICES   PREP : 10 MINUTES   COOK : 40 MINUTES

2 cups almond flour
½ cup linseed, sunflower and almond meal (LSA)
¼ cup coconut flour
2 teaspoons gluten-free baking powder
¼ teaspoon sea salt
4 free-range eggs, whisked
¼ cup cold-pressed extra-virgin coconut oil, melted
2 tablespoons apple cider vinegar
1 zucchini, grated

1   Preheat oven to 180°C and line a bread tin with baking paper.
2   In a large bowl, place almond flour, LSA, coconut flour, baking powder and salt, and stir to combine.
3   Separate eggs. Whisk whites well and add to the bowl, then add whisked yolks.
4   Add coconut oil and vinegar. Stir well, ensuring all the dry mix has taken up the liquid. Stir through the grated zucchini.
5   Scoop into the prepared tin and bake for 30–40 minutes, or until a skewer inserted into the centre comes out clean.
6   Cool in the tin, cut into 12 slices and store in an airtight container in the fridge for up to 10 days. This bread also freezes well.

MACROS   Cals : 195   CHO : 7g   P : 9g   Fat : 15g

This is one of my absolute favourite bread recipes. It's delicious toasted with grass-fed butter, is a great bread replacement in any cooked breakfast and is the ideal accompaniment to a bowl of soup. Make a loaf on Sunday and you're set for the week ahead.

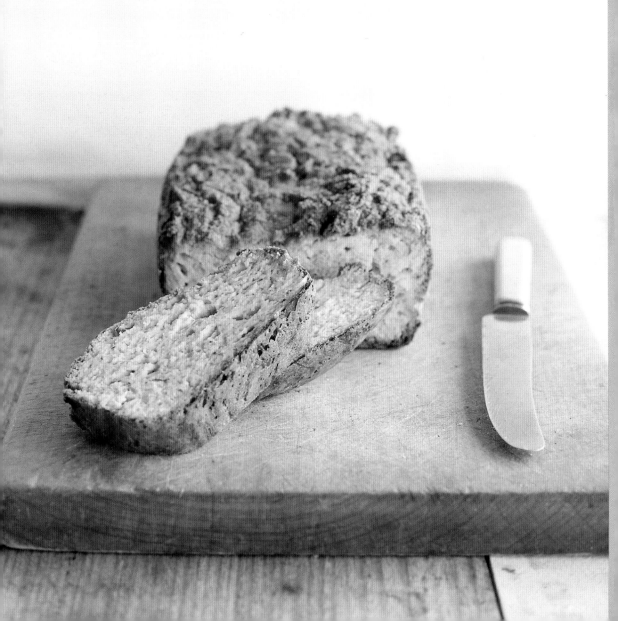

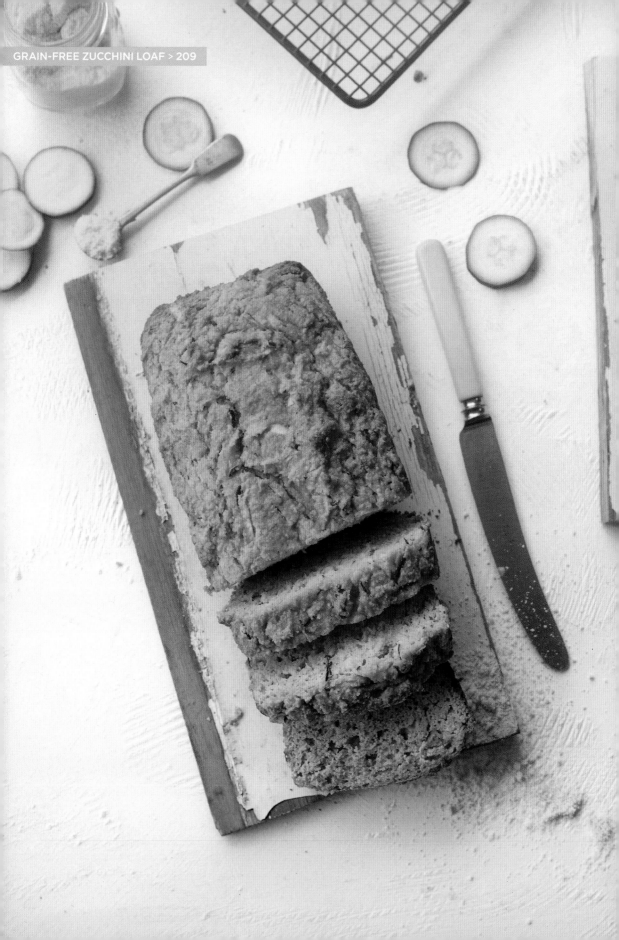

GRAIN-FREE ZUCCHINI LOAF

MAKES : 12 SLICES   PREP : 10 MINUTES   COOK : 40 MINUTES

2 cups almond meal
¼ cup buckwheat flour
2 tablespoons psyllium husks
1½ teaspoons gluten-free baking powder
¼ teaspoon sea salt
4 free-range eggs, whisked
1 tablespoon apple cider vinegar
1 tablespoon organic rice malt syrup
¼ cup cold-pressed extra-virgin coconut oil
1 zucchini, grated

1 Preheat oven to 180°C and line a bread tin with baking paper.

2 In a large bowl, place almond meal, buckwheat flour, psyllium husks, baking powder and salt, and stir to combine.

3 To the bowl add eggs, vinegar, rice malt syrup and coconut oil. Stir well, ensuring all the dry mix has taken up the liquid. Let the mixture sit for 5 minutes to allow the psyllium to go to work.

4 Add the grated zucchini and combine thoroughly.

5 Scoop into the prepared tin and bake for 35–40 minutes, or until a skewer inserted into the centre comes out clean.

6 Cool in the tin, cut into 12 slices and store in an airtight container in the fridge for up to 10 days. This bread also freezes well.

MACROS   Cals : 239   CHO : 8g   P : 9g   Fat : 20g

GLUTEN-FREE SPINACH BREAD

MAKES : 12 SLICES   PREP : 10 MINUTES   COOK : 40 MINUTES

This bread is so popular, and one of the first recipes I ever created. I love to get green vegetables into as many meals as possible, and I can't go past a slice of bread with butter, so this really is the perfect combination for me.

2½ cups almond flour
¼ teaspoon sea salt
2 teaspoons gluten-free baking powder
1½ cups finely chopped or blended spinach leaves
4 free-range eggs, whisked
¼ cup cold-pressed extra-virgin coconut oil
1 tablespoon organic rice malt syrup
1 tablespoon apple cider vinegar

1 Preheat oven to 180°C and line a bread tin with baking paper.

2 In a large bowl, place almond flour, salt and baking powder, and stir to combine.

3 Add the spinach, eggs, coconut oil, rice malt syrup and vinegar. Stir well, ensuring all the dry mix has taken up the liquid.

4 Scoop into the prepared tin and bake for 30–40 minutes, or until a skewer inserted into the centre comes out clean.

5 Cool in the tin, cut into 12 slices and store in an airtight container in the fridge for up to 10 days. This bread also freezes well.

MACROS   Cals : 223   CHO : 6g   P : 8g   Fat : 19g

SAVOURY BREAKFAST MUFFINS

MAKES : 8 MUFFINS   PREP : 15 MINUTES   COOK : 30 MINUTES

2½ cups almond or hazelnut
    meal
1 teaspoon gluten-free baking
    powder
¼ teaspoon sea salt
1 tablespoon apple cider vinegar
4 free-range eggs, whisked
½ cup grass-fed butter, melted
1 zucchini, grated
½ cup grated sweet potato
1 teaspoon cold-pressed
    extra-virgin coconut oil
2 rashers pasture-raised bacon,
    diced

1 Preheat oven to 180°C and line a muffin tray with muffin
   cases.

2 In a large bowl, place almond or hazelnut meal, baking
   powder, salt and vinegar, and stir to combine. Add the eggs,
   melted butter and grated vegies, and stir well to combine

3 Heat a small frypan over medium heat, add the oil and fry
   the bacon. Add to the bowl and combine well.

4 Transfer mixture evenly to the 8 muffin cases and bake for
   30 minutes, or until a skewer inserted into the centre comes
   out clean.

5 Allow to cool slightly before serving. Leftovers will keep in
   the fridge for 4–5 days. The muffins also freeze well.

MACROS   Cals : **353** CHO : **8g**   P : **15g** Fat : **30g**

'ON-THE-GO' MUFFINS

MAKES : 10 MUFFINS   PREP : 15 MINUTES   COOK : 25 MINUTES

The perfect breakfast when you're on the go. I always like to have a batch in the
freezer, which can be quickly toasted and topped with grass-fed butter, for a
nutrient-dense and time-efficient start to the day. These also double as a great snack.

2½ cups almond meal
1 teaspoon gluten-free baking
    powder
½ teaspoon sea salt
1 tablespoon apple cider
    vinegar
½ tablespoon cold-pressed
    extra-virgin coconut oil
2 rashers pasture-raised bacon,
    diced
4 free-range eggs, whisked
½ cup grass-fed butter, melted
1 zucchini, grated
1 cup grated pumpkin
2 tablespoons pumpkin seeds

1 Preheat oven to 180°C and line a muffin tray with muffin
   cases.

2 In a large bowl, place almond meal, baking powder, salt
   and vinegar and stir to combine.

3 Heat a small frypan over medium heat, add the oil and fry
   the bacon until crispy. Allow to cool.

4 To the bowl, add eggs and butter, mixing well to combine.
   Add the bacon and grated vegies and stir well.

5 Transfer mixture evenly to the 10 muffin cases, top with a
   smattering of pumpkin seeds and bake for 25 minutes,
   or until a skewer inserted into the centre comes out clean.

6 Serve 1–2 muffins for breakfast. Leftovers will keep in
   the fridge for 4–5 days, and also freeze well.

MACROS   Cals : **286** CHO : **7g**   P : **12g** Fat : **24g**

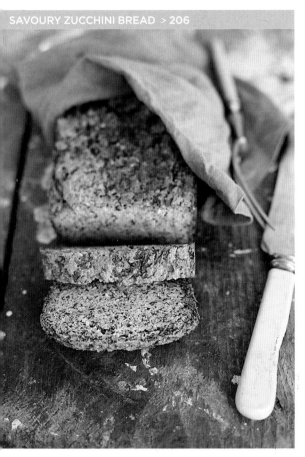

SAVOURY ZUCCHINI BREAD > 206

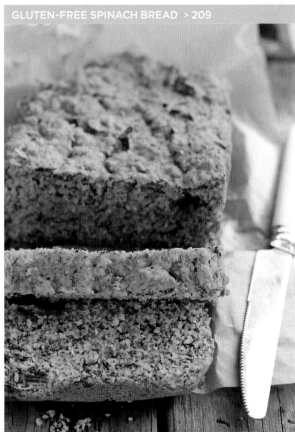

GLUTEN-FREE SPINACH BREAD > 209

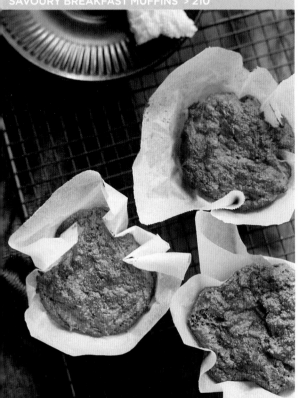

SAVOURY BREAKFAST MUFFINS > 210

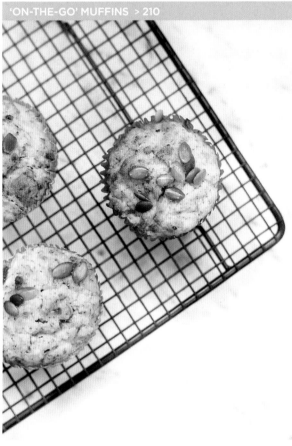

'ON-THE-GO' MUFFINS > 210

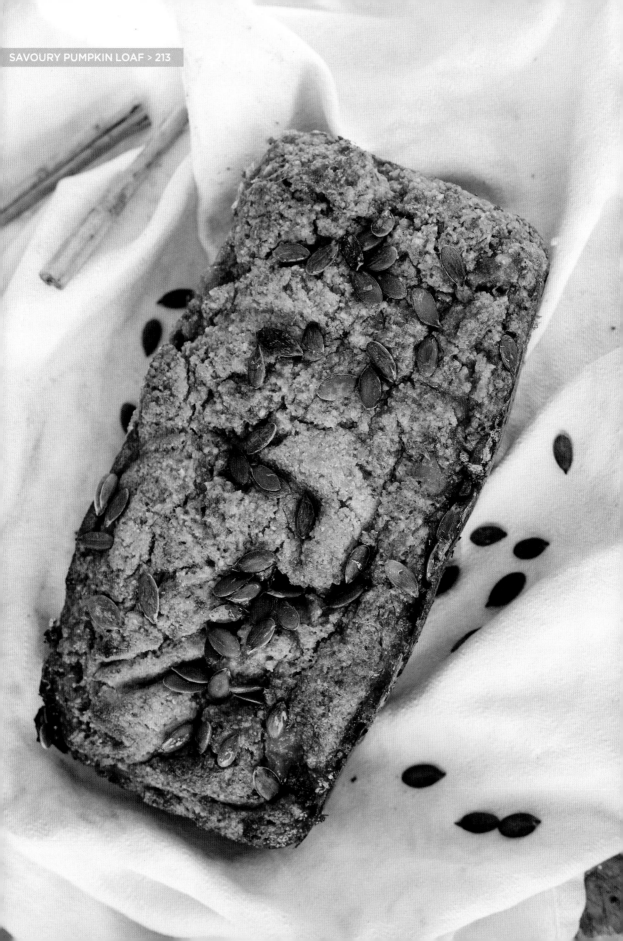

GLUTEN-FREE SAVOURY LOAF

MAKES : 10 SLICES   PREP : 15 MINUTES   COOK : 30 MINUTES

2 tablespoons chia seeds
2 cups almond meal
1 tablespoon nutritional yeast
1 zucchini, roughly chopped
1 teaspoon gluten-free baking
  powder
¼ cup cold-pressed extra-virgin
  coconut oil
½ teaspoon sea salt
1 tablespoon pumpkin seeds
⅓ cup marinated sundried
  tomatoes, drained and
  roughly chopped
⅓ cup marinated artichoke
  hearts, drained and roughly
  chopped

1 Preheat oven to 180°C and line a bread tin with baking paper.

2 Prepare the 'chia seed eggs' by combining chia seeds with
   120ml of water in a bowl. Stir well and allow to rest for
   15 minutes.

3 Process almond meal, nutritional yeast, zucchini, baking
   powder, coconut oil and salt in a food processor or blender.
   Add 'chia eggs' and blend until well combined.

4 Add pumpkin seeds, sundried tomatoes and artichoke
   hearts, and pulse until just combined.

5 Scoop into the prepared tin and bake for 20–25 minutes,
   or until golden on top and a skewer inserted into the centre
   comes out clean.

6 Cool in the tin, cut into 10 slices and store in an airtight
   container in the fridge for up to 10 days. This loaf also
   freezes well.

MACROS   Cals : **440**   CHO : **16g**   P : **13g**   Fat : **36g**

SAVOURY PUMPKIN LOAF

MAKES : 10 SLICES   PREP : 10 MINUTES   COOK : 40 MINUTES

2½ cups almond flour
¼ teaspoon sea salt
2 teaspoons gluten-free baking
  powder
1 cup grated pumpkin
4 free-range eggs, whisked
¼ cup cold-pressed extra-virgin
  coconut oil, melted
1 tablespoon organic rice malt
  syrup
1 tablespoon apple cider
  vinegar

1 Preheat oven to 180°C and line a bread tin with baking
   paper.

2 In a large bowl, place almond flour, salt and baking powder,
   and stir to combine.

3 Add the pumpkin, eggs, coconut oil, rice malt syrup and
   vinegar. Stir well, ensuring all the dry mix has taken up the
   liquid.

4 Scoop into the prepared tin and bake for 30–40 minutes,
   or until a skewer inserted into the centre comes out clean.

5 Cool in the tin, cut into 10 slices and store in an airtight
   container in the fridge for up to 10 days. This loaf also
   freezes well.

MACROS   Cals : **270**   CHO : **8g**   P : **10g**   Fat : **23g**

RASPBERRY & CHIA BREAD

MAKES : 10 SLICES   PREP : 10 MINUTES   COOK : 40 MINUTES

This is a real treat! Being egg free, it's a great one to include whenever you are having a break from eggs, and the perfect recipe to share with your vegan friends. Serve with lashings of grass-fed butter or almond butter, depending on your preference.

4 tablespoons chia seeds
2½ cups almond flour
1 tablespoon buckwheat flour
1 teaspoon cinnamon
1 teaspoon gluten-free baking powder
¼ teaspoon sea salt
1 teaspoon organic vanilla extract
¼ cup cold-pressed extra-virgin coconut oil, melted
¼ cup organic rice malt syrup
1 tablespoon apple cider vinegar
1 cup raspberries
¼ cup unsweetened coconut flakes

1   Preheat oven to 180°C and line a bread tin with baking paper.

2   Prepare 'chia seed eggs' by combining chia seeds with 240ml water in a bowl. Stir well and allow to rest for 15 minutes.

3   Meanwhile, in a large bowl, place flours, cinnamon, baking powder and salt, and stir to combine.

4   Add 'chia eggs', vanilla extract, coconut oil, rice malt syrup and vinegar, and mix thoroughly.

5   Carefully fold in raspberries and coconut. If the mixture is very thick, add ½ cup water, mix thoroughly and allow to sit for 15 minutes.

6   Scoop into the prepared tin and bake for 30–40 minutes, or until a skewer inserted into the centre comes out clean.

7   Cool in the tin, cut into 10 slices and store in an airtight container in the fridge for up to 10 days. This bread also freezes well.

MACROS   Cals : **334** CHO : **27g** P : **7g**   Fat : **24g**

SNACKS

Snacking is optional with a well-balanced LCHF approach, and should really only be necessary when a longer meal-to-meal window arises. The following are my go-to LCHF snacks. Remember to keep it simple and when you build your meals the LCHF way, you will find yourself snacking far less.

NUT-FREE TRAIL MIX

MAKES : 8 SERVES   PREP : 5 MINUTES

This is one of my most popular lunchbox-friendly snacks. I love to add raw dark chocolate, free of refined sugar. The recipe doubles as a dessert.

½ cup sunflower seeds
½ cup pumpkin seeds
45g cacao nibs (or your
    favourite dark chocolate,
    roughly chopped)
30g shredded coconut
½ teaspoon cinnamon
¼ teaspoon sea salt

Combine all the ingredients in a large bowl, share out and enjoy.

MACROS   Cals : 171   CHO : 6g   P : 12g   Fat : 14g

TWO BOILED EGGS

SERVES Ⓕ Ⓜ 1   PREP : 5 MINUTES   COOK : 5 MINUTES

2 free-range eggs

Bring a small saucepan of water to the boil. Carefully add eggs and reduce heat to a simmer. Cook for 4–5 minutes. Run under cold water before peeling.

MACROS   Cals : 143   CHO : 1g   P : 13g   Fat : 10g

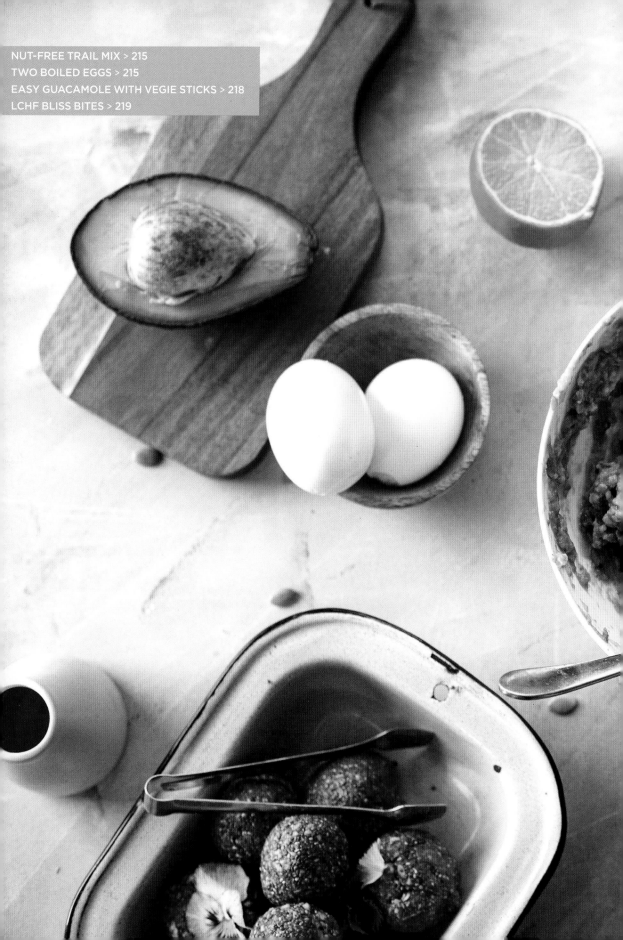

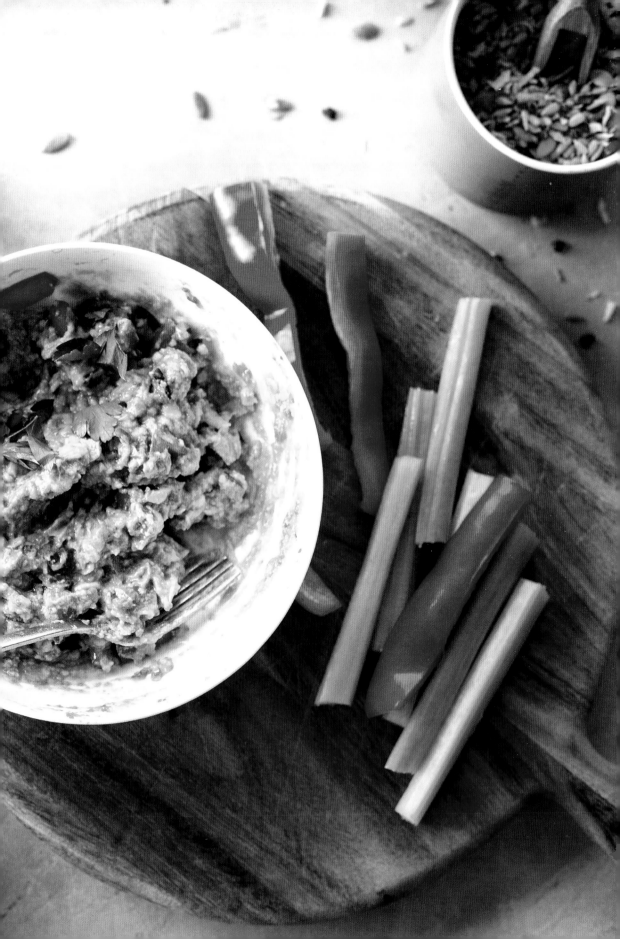

'BUILD YOUR OWN' EGG CUPS

MAKES : 12   PREP : 10 MINUTES   COOK : 10 MINUTES

Packed full of protein, these are fantastic snacks for when you're on the go. Some of my favourite combinations are: bacon, mushroom and sundried tomatoes; sweet potato, broccolini and chilli; and mushroom, sundried tomato, capsicum, chives and feta. You are limited only by your imagination with these.

½ tablespoon cold-pressed extra-virgin coconut oil, melted
12 free-range eggs
sea salt and pepper, to taste
toppings of your choice, such as bacon, mushroom, sundried tomatoes, sweet potato, broccolini, capsicum, chives
goat's feta, optional

1   Preheat oven to 150°C and, using the coconut oil, lightly grease a 12-hole muffin tray.

2   Whisk eggs in a large bowl and season with salt and pepper to taste. Pour into muffin holes until three-quarters full.

3   Finely chop topping ingredients and add a handful to each muffin hole. If using feta, add a small cube to each.

4   Bake for 10 minutes, or until cooked through. Your egg cups should increase in size and then settle once removed from the oven and cooled. Store in an airtight container in the fridge for up to 5 days.

MACROS   Cals : **109**   CHO : **1g**   P : **8g**   Fat : **7g**

EASY GUACAMOLE WITH VEGIE STICKS

SERVES Ⓕ Ⓜ 4 / 2   PREP : 10 MINUTES

2 avocados, diced
2 tomatoes, diced
1 red onion, chopped
2 handfuls coriander, finely chopped
1 lime, juiced
2 tablespoons extra-virgin olive oil
4 cups chopped vegetables such as carrot, celery, capsicum, cucumber / 2 cups chopped vegetables such as carrot, celery, capsicum, cucumber

1   Place avocado, tomato, onion and coriander in a bowl. Add lime juice and olive oil and roughly crush the ingredients with the back of a fork. Serve with 1 cup of your favourite chopped vegetables.

2   This guacamole can be stored in an airtight container in the fridge for up to 5 days.

Ⓕ MACROS Cals : **239**   CHO : **20g**   P : **3g**   Fat : **18g**
Ⓜ MACROS Cals : **478**   CHO : **41g**   P : **6g**   Fat : **36g**

LCHF BLISS BITES

MAKES : 10   PREP : 20 MINUTES

My LCHF Bliss Bites are everyone's favourite! Sweetened only with stevia, they are much lower in carbohydrates than most bliss bites or protein balls, and the absence of dates makes them extremely low fructose as well. These are great as a snack during a long hike, run or bike ride.

1 tablespoon chia seeds
250g cashews
1 scoop vanilla or chocolate grass-fed whey protein powder
2 tablespoons raw cacao
1–1½ tablespoons stevia, depending on desired sweetness
1 tablespoon cinnamon
¼ cup cold-pressed extra-virgin coconut oil, melted
extra chia seeds and/or protein powder, for coating

1   Soak chia seeds in ¼ cup of water for 10 minutes.

2   In a large bowl, place cashews, protein powder, cacao, stevia and cinnamon. Add melted coconut oil and stir well.

3   Add the soaked chia seeds and stir to combine.

4   Using an ice-cream scoop or spoon, form the mixture into 8 balls that each sit nicely in the palm of your hand. (To prevent them sticking, add a touch of oil to your hands prior to doing so).

5   Sprinkle the extra chia seeds and/or protein powder, and chill in the fridge before serving. Store in an airtight container in the fridge for up to 10 days.

MACROS   Cals : **163**   CHO : **8g**   P : **7g**   Fat : **13g**

TREATS

Going LCHF definitely doesn't mean that you have to miss out. My general advice is to enjoy no more than two treats per week, but this of course depends on your starting point, your current metabolic state, and your specific health or body compositional goals.

MINTY FAT BOMB

MAKES : 12   PREP : 5 MINUTES

1 cup cold-pressed extra-virgin coconut oil
½ cup raw cacao
½ teaspoon vanilla bean powder
pinch of sea salt
1–2 drops organic peppermint essential oil
5 drops liquid stevia

1 Process all the ingredients together in a food processor or blender until the mixture is smooth and creamy.
2 Pour into ice-cube trays, or similar sized silicone moulds, and freeze.
3 Once frozen, pop the fat bombs out of the moulds and store them in the freezer.

MACROS   Cals : 175   CHO : 2g   P : 1g   Fat : 19g

CHOC ALMOND BUTTER CUPS

SERVES Ⓕ Ⓜ 6   PREP : 20 MINUTES

BOTTOM LAYER
½ cup almond butter
¼ cup cold-pressed extra-virgin coconut oil, melted
¼ teaspoon cinnamon

TOP LAYER
¼ cup raw cacao
¼ cup cold-pressed extra-virgin coconut oil, melted
½ teaspoon raw honey
pinch of sea salt

1 Line a 6-hole muffin pan with muffin cases.
2 To make the bottom layer of the cups, place all the ingredients in a bowl and stir to combine. Spoon into the muffin cases and place in the fridge for 10 minutes to firm.
3 To make the top layer, place all the ingredients in a bowl and whisk well to combine. Spoon over the bottom layer and return to the fridge for a further 10 minutes to firm.
4 Best eaten straight out of the fridge or freezer, where they can be stored.

MACROS   Cals : 335   CHO : 8g   P : 7g   Fat : 31g

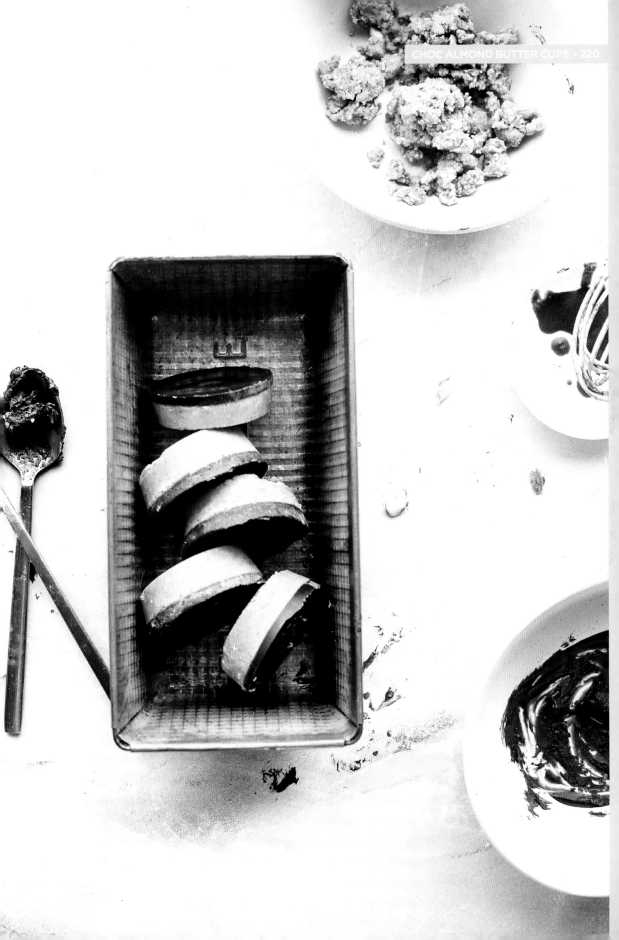

CHOC ALMOND BUTTER CUPS > 220

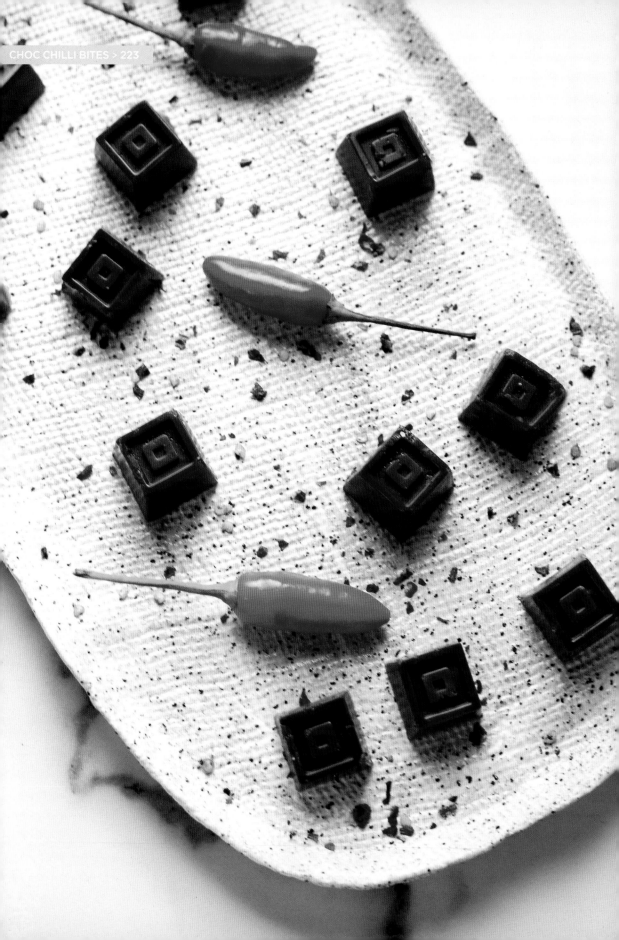

CHOC CHILLI BITES

MAKES : 12   PREP : 5 MINUTES   COOK : 5 MINUTES + FREEZING TIME

½ cup cold-pressed extra-virgin coconut oil
2 tablespoons raw cacao
1–2 tablespoons organic rice malt syrup, depending on desired sweetness
1–2 teaspoons chilli flakes, depending on how much bite you like
¼ teaspoon sea salt

1 Melt coconut oil in a small saucepan over low heat. Add all the remaining ingredients and stir well to combine.

2 Pour into ice-cube trays, or similar sized silicone moulds, and freeze.

3 Once frozen, pop the chilli bites out of the moulds and store them in the freezer.

MACROS   Cals : 142   CHO : 3g   P : 0g   Fat : 14g

LCHF RASPBERRY BOUNTY BARS

SERVES (F)(M) 10   PREP : 30 MINUTES   FREEZE : 4½ HOURS

Tell me you didn't love a Bounty Bar during your childhood! My LCHF version has a raspberry twist on the original, and in my opinion is even more delicious. This recipe does have a few more steps than my usual recipes, but it's very much worth the time investment for a special occasion.

COCONUT LAYER
1 cup shredded coconut
¼ cup coconut cream
½ teaspoon organic vanilla extract
1 tablespoon cold-pressed extra-virgin coconut oil, melted
pinch of sea salt

RASPBERRY LAYER
1 cup shredded coconut
¼ cup coconut cream
1 tablespoon cold-pressed extra-virgin coconut oil, melted
150g raspberries
pinch of sea salt

CHOCOLATE LAYER
¼ cup raw cacao
¼ cup cold-pressed extra-virgin coconut oil, melted
½ teaspoon raw honey
pinch of sea salt

1 Line a 20cm square baking tin with baking paper.

2 To make the coconut layer: Place all the ingredients in a food processor or blender and pulse until well combined. Transfer to the baking tin and press down to ensure the mixture is evenly and tightly packed. Place in the freezer for 10 minutes while you make the raspberry layer.

3 To make the raspberry layer: Place all the ingredients in a food processor or blender and pulse until well combined. If you'd like the raspberry layer to be a little chunkier, add raspberries after the other ingredients are combined and pulse once or twice. Place on top of the coconut layer and press down evenly. Use your fingers or the back of a spoon to smooth the top. Place in the freezer for 4 hours, or until set.

4 To make the chocolate layer: Place all the ingredients in a bowl and whisk well to combine.

5 Remove the tray from the freezer and slice into 10 bars. Coat each bar in chocolate and place in the fridge to firm.

MACROS   Cals : 253   CHO : 10g   P : 2g   Fat : 23g

LAYERED SEED FAT BOMBS

SERVES Ⓕ Ⓜ 6   PREP : 15 MINUTES

SUNFLOWER SEED LAYER
¼ cup cold-pressed extra-virgin
   coconut oil, melted
¼ cup sunflower seed butter
pinch of sea salt

PUMPKIN SEED LAYER
¼ cup cold-pressed extra-virgin
   coconut oil, melted
¼ cup pumpkin seed butter
pinch of sea salt

1 Line a 6-hole muffin pan with muffin cases.

2 To make the sunflower seed layer, place all the ingredients in a bowl and stir well to combine. Spoon into the muffin cases and place in the fridge for 10 minutes to firm.

3 To make the pumpkin seed layer, place all the ingredients in a bowl and stir well to combine. Spoon onto the sunflower seed layer and place in the freezer for 5 minutes to firm.

4 Best eaten straight from the fridge or freezer, where they can be stored.

MACROS   Cals : **273**   CHO : **4g**   P : **8g**   Fat : **28g**

CLEAN BERRY ICE-CREAM

SERVES Ⓕ Ⓜ 4   PREP : 5 MINUTES   FREEZE : 2 HOURS

400ml coconut cream
1 cup blueberries
1 tablespoon cold-pressed
   extra-virgin coconut oil
1 teaspoon organic rice
   malt syrup
fresh mint, to garnish

1 Place all the ingredients (except mint) in a high-powered blender and start blending on low, gradually increasing to high. Blend until creamy. Make sure you don't blend on high for too long, as this acts as a heating function.

2 Pour into a shallow dish and freeze for 2 hours.

3 Serve into bowls using a large ice-cream scoop, top with mint and enjoy. Keep leftovers well-sealed in the freezer and use within a few days.

MACROS   Cals : **235**   CHO : **8g**   P : **2g**   Fat : **24g**

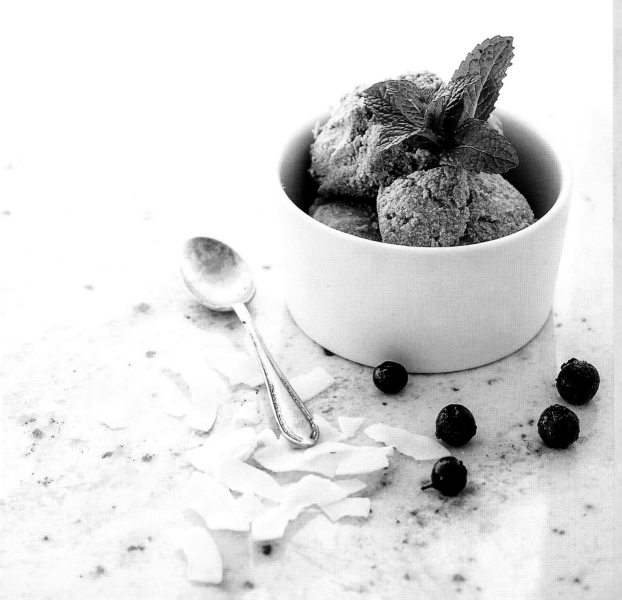

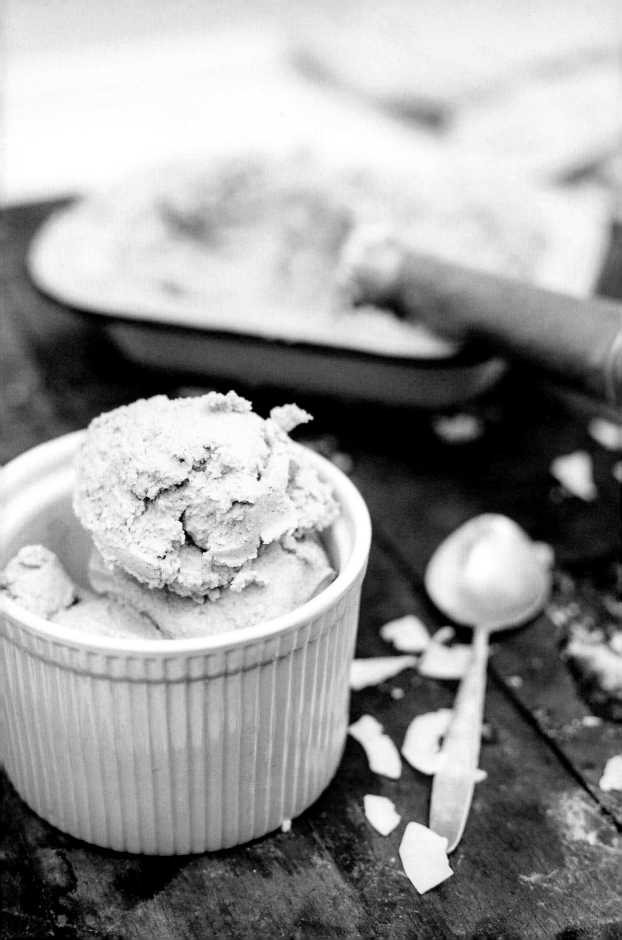

SUPER-EASY COCONUT ICE-CREAM

SERVES Ⓕ Ⓜ 4   PREP : 5 MINUTES   FREEZE : 2 HOURS

I frequently make this when the weather warms up, but it's a simple and versatile treat you can enjoy any time. Just five ingredients and five minutes of prep time – it's easy to see why this is a favourite!

400ml coconut cream
¼ cup coconut butter
1 teaspoon cinnamon
1 teaspoon stevia
1 tablespoon organic rice
   malt syrup

1 Place all the ingredients in a high-powered blender and start blending on low, gradually increasing to high. Blend until creamy. Make sure you don't blend on high for too long, as this acts as a heating function.

2 Pour into a shallow dish and freeze for 2 hours.

3 Serve into bowls using a large ice-cream scoop, and enjoy. Keep leftovers well-sealed in the freezer and use within a few days.

MACROS   Cals : 348   CHO : 16g   P : 4g   Fat : 32g

These LCHF drinks and smoothies will provide you with some simple substitutes for your current choices. I personally love smoothies – they're a time-efficient and delicious way to sneak in a few extra vegetables!

MELROSE MCT COFFEE

SERVES (F) (M) 1   PREP : 5 MINUTES

You're going to love this simple MCT coffee for clean, instant energy, fat burning, increased mental output and satiety. It's a perfect breakfast replacement and the best pre-workout drink there is!

¼–⅓ cup organic coffee beans, ground
1 tablespoon grass-fed unsalted butter or ghee
1 teaspoon MCT oil

1 Make a standard espresso using a coffee machine, or by your preferred method.
2 Add hot water to a blender to preheat it, then tip out the water.
3 Add coffee, butter or ghee and MCT oil, and blend for 20–30 seconds or until creamy and well combined.

MACROS   Cals : 150   CHO : 0g   P : 0g   Fat : 19g

ANTI-INFLAMMATORY MCT COFFEE

SERVES (F) (M) 1   PREP : 5 MINUTES

¼–⅓ cup organic coffee beans, ground
1 tablespoon grass-fed unsalted butter or ghee
1 teaspoon MCT oil
1 teaspoon turmeric powder

1 Make a standard espresso using a coffee machine, or by your preferred method.
2 Add hot water to a blender to preheat it, then tip out the water.
3 Add coffee, butter or ghee, MCT oil and turmeric, and blend for 20–30 seconds or until creamy and well combined.

MACROS   Cals : 150   CHO : 0g   P : 0g   Fat : 19g

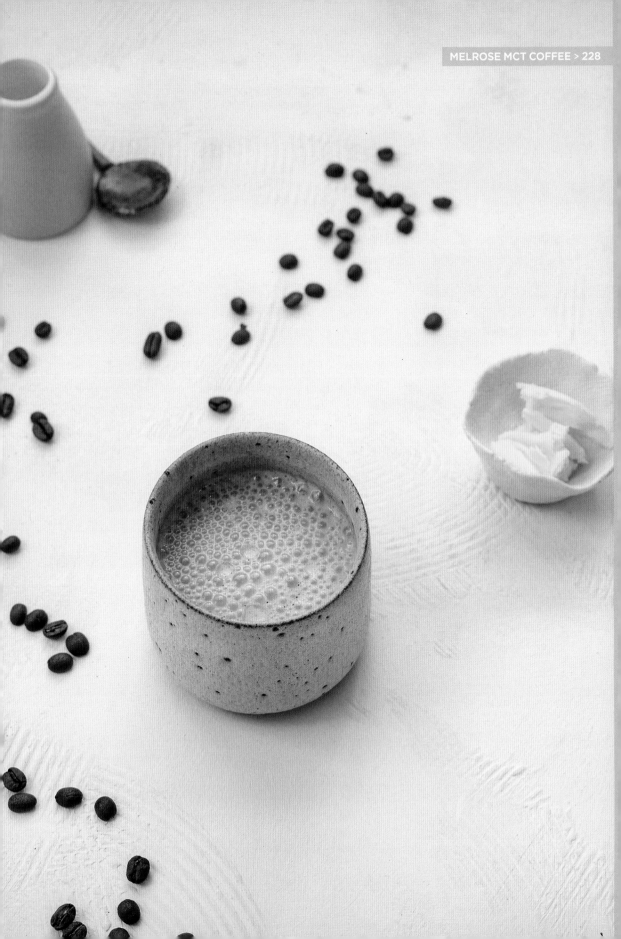

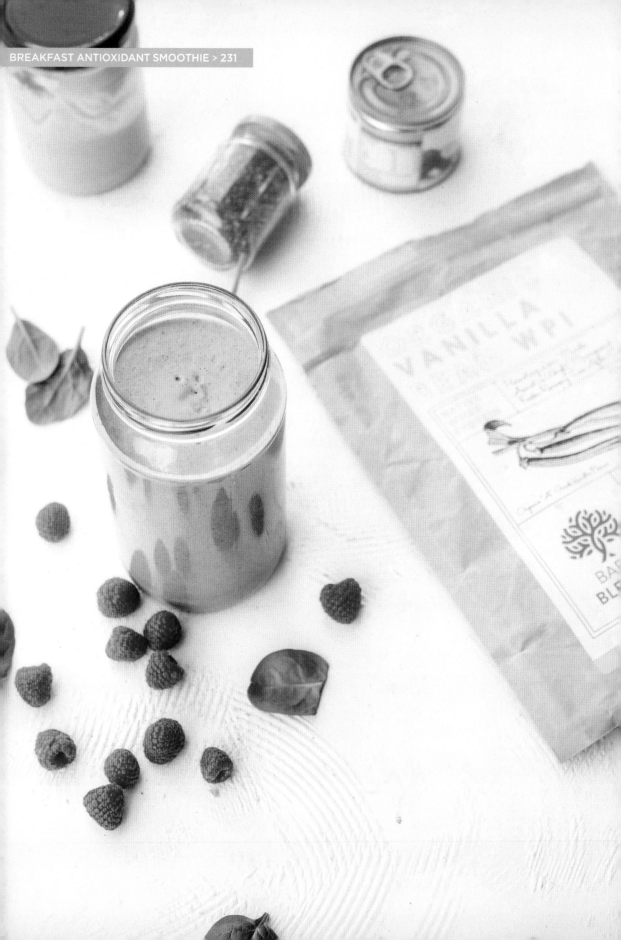

HORMONAL-BALANCING MCT COFFEE

SERVES (F)(M) 1   PREP : 5 MINUTES

The addition of maca powder to your MCT coffee not only gives it a nice nutty flavour but nourishes your master glands – the hypothalamus and the pituitary gland – which helps to balance your hormones.

¼–⅓ cup organic coffee beans, ground
1 tablespoon grass-fed unsalted butter or ghee
1 teaspoon MCT oil
1 teaspoon maca powder

1 Make a standard espresso using a coffee machine, or by your preferred method.
2 Add hot water to a blender to preheat it, then tip out the water.
3 Add coffee, butter or ghee, MCT oil and maca powder, and blend for 20–30 seconds or until creamy and well combined.

MACROS   Cals : 150   CHO : 0g   P : 0g   Fat : 19g

BREAKFAST ANTIOXIDANT SMOOTHIE #1

SERVES (F)(M) 1   PREP : 15 MINUTES

This is my favourite mid-week breakfast. If you're new to LCHF, you may need to add half a banana to sweeten it, but remember your tastebuds will quickly change as you decrease your reliance on refined carbohydrates and sugars.

1 teaspoon chia seeds
100ml coconut cream /
    150ml coconut cream
¼ avocado / ½ avocado
1 tablespoon cashew butter
20g spinach leaves
½ cup raspberries / 1 cup
    raspberries
1 teaspoon cinnamon
2 teaspoons cold-pressed extra-virgin coconut oil or MCT oil
1 scoop vanilla or chocolate grass-fed whey protein powder
⅓–1 tray ice

1 Place chia seeds and 1 cup of water in a blender and let sit for 5 minutes for the chia seeds to go to work.
2 Add coconut cream, avocado, cashew butter, spinach, raspberries, cinnamon and oil, and blend well.
3 Add protein powder and ice, and blend until thick but smooth. Add more ice for a thicker smoothie.
4 Pour into a jar and transport with you as required. Enjoy.

(F) MACROS Cals : 701   CHO : 22g   P : 38g   Fat : 46g
(M) MACROS Cals : 701   CHO : 34g   P : 40g   Fat : 62g

This really is a well-balanced meal in a jar, and the perfectly portable way to break your overnight fast. The addition of zucchini is a great way to sneak in extra greens, and you won't even taste it!

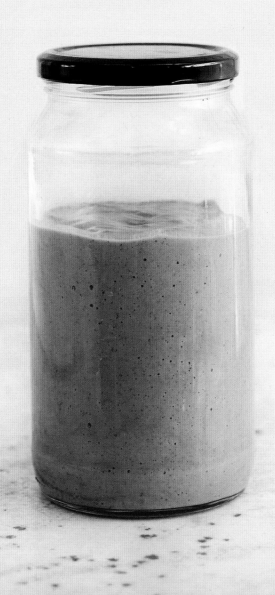

BREAKFAST ANTIOXIDANT SMOOTHIE #2

SERVES (F)(M) 1   PREP : 15 MINUTES

1 teaspoon chia seeds
100ml coconut cream /
   150ml coconut cream
½ avocado
20g kale, roughly chopped
½ cup raspberries / 1 cup
   raspberries
1 teaspoon cinnamon
1 scoop vanilla or chocolate
   grass-fed whey protein
   powder
⅓–1 tray ice

1 Place chia seeds and 1 cup of water in a blender and let
   sit for 5 minutes for the chia seeds to go to work.

2 Add coconut cream, avocado, kale, raspberries and
   cinnamon, and blend well.

3 Add protein powder and ice, and blend until thick but
   smooth. Add more ice for a thicker smoothie.

4 Pour into a jar and transport with you as required. Enjoy.

(F) MACROS   Cals : **588**   CHO : **21g**   P : **36g**   Fat : **34g**
(M) MACROS   Cals : **728**   CHO : **30g**   P : **38g**   Fat : **41g**

MEAL IN A JAR

SERVES (F)(M) 1   PREP : 15 MINUTES

1 teaspoon chia seeds /
   1 tablespoon chia seeds
65ml coconut cream /
   125ml coconut cream
½ avocado
½ small banana
20g spinach leaves
1 zucchini, roughly chopped
¼ cup blueberries, fresh or
   frozen / ½ cup blueberries,
   fresh or frozen
¼ teaspoon cinnamon
1 tablespoon cold-pressed
   extra-virgin coconut oil
2 tablespoons vanilla or
   chocolate grass-fed whey
   protein powder
⅓–1 tray ice

1 Place chia seeds and 1 cup of water in a blender and let
   sit for 5 minutes for the chia seeds to go to work.

2 Add coconut cream, avocado, banana, spinach, zucchini,
   blueberries, cinnamon and oil, and blend well.

3 Add protein powder and ice, and blend until thick but
   smooth. Add more ice for a thicker smoothie.

4 Pour into a jar and transport with you as required. Enjoy.

(F) MACROS   Cals : **677**   CHO : **41g**   P : **36g**   Fat : **33g**
(M) MACROS   Cals : **909**   CHO : **47g**   P : **40g**   Fat : **64g**

LOWER-CARB SMOOTHIE BOWL

SERVES (F) (M) 1   PREP : 15 MINUTES

Smoothie bowls are notoriously high in carbohydrates and often packed with high-sugar fruits such as bananas and dates. My smoothie bowl is just as delicious as a shop-bought version, with a fraction of the carbs. The addition of gelatin is fantastic for gut healing, immune support and skin integrity.

250ml unsweetened nut milk
1 tablespoon chia seeds
½ cup frozen raspberries
½ cup frozen blueberries
1 tablespoon grass-fed
    whey protein powder /
    2 tablespoons grass-fed
    whey protein powder
1 tablespoon nut butter
20g spinach leaves
1 teaspoon grass-fed gelatin
¼ teaspoon cinnamon

TO SERVE
1 teaspoon unsweetened
    coconut flakes / 1 tablespoon
    unsweetened coconut flakes
1 teaspoon cacao nibs /
    1 tablespoon cacao nibs
1 tablespoon goji berries

1   Place nut milk and chia seeds in a blender and let sit for 5 minutes for the chia seeds to go to work.

2   Add remaining smoothie ingredients to the blender and blend until creamy and thick. If the consistency is too thick, slowly blend in a little extra nut milk.

3   Spoon the mixture into a bowl and top with coconut flakes, cacao nibs and goji berries.

(F) MACROS   Cals : **433**   CHO : **46g**   P : **11g**   Fat : **27g**
(M) MACROS   Cals : **735**   CHO : **54g**   P : **41g**   Fat : **44g**

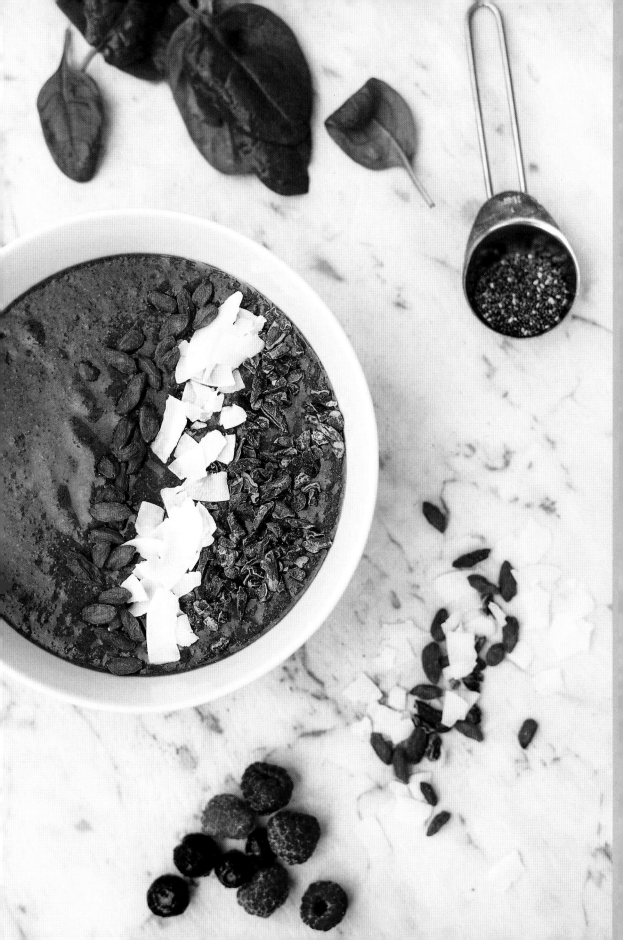

A smoothie without fruit? You won't believe how good this tastes! I even enjoy this for lunch if I've eaten out for breakfast that morning. If you don't have access to a blender during the day, simply make it before you leave for work in the morning.

GREEN MACHINE SMOOTHIE

SERVES Ⓕ Ⓜ 1   PREP : 15 MINUTES

250ml unsweetened
   almond milk
1 tablespoon chia seeds
20g spinach leaves
1 tablespoon almond butter
1 tablespoon cashews
1 tablespoon cold-pressed
   extra-virgin coconut oil
½ avocado
1 tablespoon grass-fed
   whey protein powder /
   2 tablespoons grass-fed
   whey protein powder
¼ teaspoon cinnamon
½ teaspoon organic vanilla
   extract
1 tray ice

1   Place almond milk and chia seeds in a blender and let sit
    for 15 minutes for the chia seeds to go to work.

2   Add remaining ingredients to the blender and blend until
    smooth or your preferred consistency.

Ⓕ MACROS   Cals : 501   CHO : 24g   P : 36g   Fat : 38g
Ⓜ MACROS   Cals : 719   CHO : 24g   P : 37g   Fat : 55g

MIXED BERRY & TAHINI SMOOTHIE

SERVES Ⓕ Ⓜ 1   PREP : 15 MINUTES

Tahini is one of my favourite ingredients. It's a great natural source of calcium and
a 20 per cent complete protein, making it a higher protein source than most nuts
and seeds.

1 tablespoon chia seeds
70ml coconut cream /
   100ml coconut cream
150g mixed berries, frozen
1 tablespoon tahini
1 cup spinach leaves
1 tablespoon grass-fed
   whey protein powder /
   2 tablespoons grass-fed
   whey protein powder
½ lemon, zested and juiced
1 cup ice, optional

1   Place chia seeds and 1 cup of water in a blender and let
    sit for 15 minutes for the chia seeds to go to work.

2   Add remaining ingredients, excluding the ice, and blend
    until smooth or your preferred consistency. If desired, add
    the ice and blend for a further minute.

Ⓕ MACROS   Cals : 569   CHO : 29g   P : 38g   Fat : 35g
Ⓜ MACROS   Cals : 767   CHO : 31g   P : 67g   Fat : 44g

BLUEBERRY & MACADAMIA SMOOTHIE

SERVES (F) (M) 1   PREP : 15 MINUTES

1 tablespoon chia seeds
1 cup coconut milk
1 cup frozen blueberries
¼ cup macadamias /
  ½ cup macadamias
¼ avocado / ½ avocado
½ teaspoon cinnamon
¼ teaspoon sea salt
1 cup ice, optional

1 Place chia seeds and coconut milk in a blender and let sit
   for 5 minutes for the chia seeds to go to work.

2 Add remaining ingredients, excluding the ice, and blend
   until smooth or your preferred consistency. If desired, add
   the ice and blend for a further minute.

(F) MACROS   Cals : 503   CHO : 37g   P : 9g   Fat : 39g
(M) MACROS   Cals : 801   CHO : 44g   P : 11g   Fat : 70g

IMMUNE-BOOSTING SMOOTHIE BOWL

SERVES (F) (M) 1   PREP : 15 MINUTES

125ml unsweetened
  almond milk
1 tablespoon chia seeds
1 cup frozen blueberries
1 tablespoon grass-fed
  whey protein powder /
  2 tablespoons grass-fed
  whey protein powder
1 tablespoon cashews
1 tablespoon almond butter
½ lemon, zested and juiced
½ teaspoon cinnamon
1 tablespoon coconut cream /
  2 tablespoons coconut cream
pinch of sea salt

TO SERVE
1 teaspoon unsweetened
  coconut flakes
1 tablespoon pumpkin seeds

1 Place almond milk and chia seeds in a blender and let
   sit for 15 minutes for the chia seeds to go to work.

2 Add remaining smoothie ingredients and blend until
   smooth or your preferred consistency.

3 Spoon the mixture into a bowl and top with coconut
   flakes and pumpkin seeds.

(F) MACROS   Cals : 514   CHO : 44g   P : 24g   Fat : 23g
(M) MACROS   Cals : 663   CHO : 55g   P : 43g   Fat : 35g

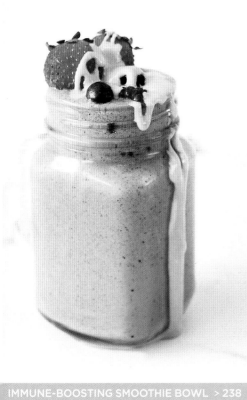

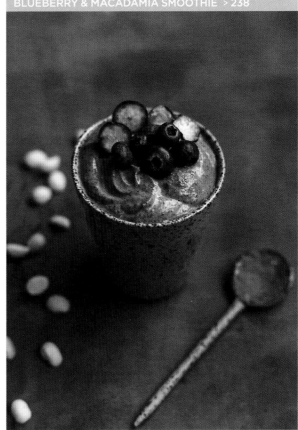

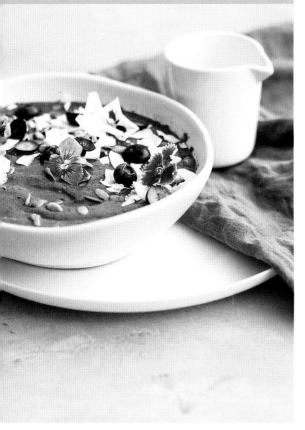

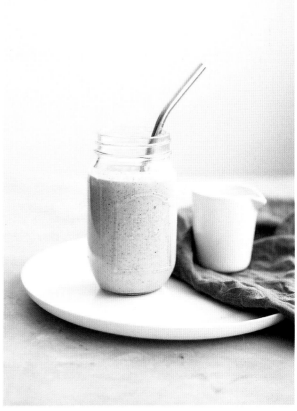

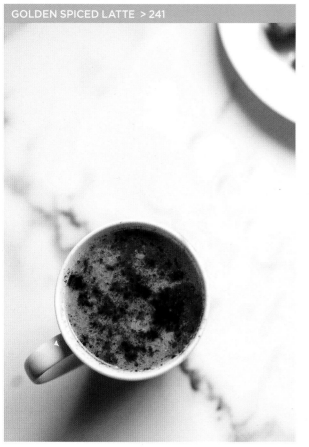

GOLDEN SPICED LATTE > 241

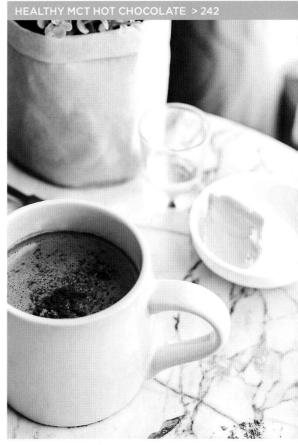

HEALTHY MCT HOT CHOCOLATE > 242

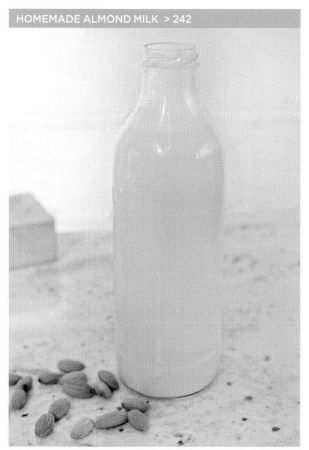

HOMEMADE ALMOND MILK > 242

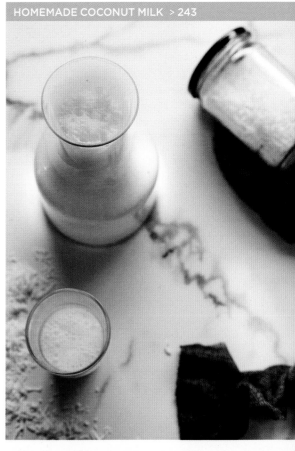

HOMEMADE COCONUT MILK > 243

MACA MAGIC SMOOTHIE

SERVES (F) (M) 1   PREP : 15 MINUTES

½ cup coconut milk
1 teaspoon chia seeds /
   1 tablespoon chia seeds
1 tablespoon pumpkin seeds
½ banana, frozen
1 tablespoon tahini /
   2 tablespoons tahini
20g kale, roughly chopped
1 teaspoon cinnamon
1 teaspoon maca powder
1 tablespoon grass-fed whey
   protein powder
½–1 tray ice

1 Place water, coconut milk and chia seeds in a blender and
   let sit for 15 minutes for the chia seeds to go to work.

2 Add remaining ingredients, excluding the ice, to the blender
   and blend until smooth or your preferred consistency. If
   desired, add the ice and blend for a further minute.

(F) MACROS   Cals : 501   CHO : 38g   P : 45g   Fat : 23g
(M) MACROS   Cals : 671   CHO : 44g   P : 52g   Fat : 36g

GOLDEN SPICED LATTE

SERVES (F) (M) 4   PREP : 5 MINUTES   COOK : 5 MINUTES

4 cups unsweetened
   coconut milk
4 teaspoons cold-pressed
   extra-virgin coconut oil
4 teaspoons turmeric powder
3 teaspoons ground ginger
3 teaspoons cinnamon
1 teaspoon nutmeg
½ teaspoon cayenne pepper
1 vanilla pod, scraped
2 tablespoons organic rice malt
   syrup, optional
pinch of sea salt
extra cinnamon, for serving

1 Place all the ingredients (except the extra cinnamon) in
   a saucepan and stir over medium heat until warmed to
   your liking.

2 Serve in mugs and sprinkle with extra cinnamon.

MACROS   Cals : 154   CHO : 17g   P : 0g   Fat : 9g

HEALTHY MCT HOT CHOCOLATE

SERVES (F)(M) 1   PREP : 10 MINUTES

This is a decadent drink that I love to consume when my lunch-to-dinner eating window is longer than five hours. The perfect cravings buster!

1 heaped teaspoon raw cacao
80ml boiling water, plus hot
**   water to preheat blender**
1 tablespoon grass-fed ghee
1 tablespoon MCT oil

1 Add hot water to a blender to preheat it, then tip out the water.

2 Add cacao, 80ml of boiling water, ghee and MCT oil. Blend for 10–20 seconds, or until creamy and well combined.

MACROS   Cals : 269 CHO : 2g   P : 2g   Fat : 28g

HOMEMADE ALMOND MILK

SERVES (F)(M) 3   PREP : 10 MINUTES + 6 HOURS SOAKING

Store-bought almond milk is often full of additives, including sugar and/or refined seed oils. Making your own is not only better for your health but also your wallet.

1 cup raw almonds
1 tablespoon organic rice malt
**   syrup**
1 tablespoon cinnamon

1 Soak almonds for at least 6 hours in 1 cup of filtered water. Drain and rinse.

2 Place almonds and 4 cups of filtered water in a blender or food processor and blend until well combined.

3 Add rice malt syrup and cinnamon and blend again, ensuring ingredients are well combined.

4 Pour through a fine-meshed strainer lined with cheesecloth into a large bowl. I cover mine and let it sit overnight to ensure the maximum liquid yield. You should get 600ml or more.

5 Pour almond milk into a tightly sealed bottle and store in the fridge for up to a week.

MACROS   Cals : 319   CHO : 15g   P : 11g   Fat : 24g

HOMEMADE COCONUT MILK

SERVES Ⓕ Ⓜ 3   PREP : 10 MINUTES + OVERNIGHT SOAKING

1 cup unsweetened coconut
flakes

OPTIONAL

1 tablespoon organic rice malt
syrup

1 tablespoon cinnamon

1 Soak coconut overnight in 1 cup of filtered water.

2 Place the entire soaked mix, plus 4 cups of filtered water, in
a blender or food processor and blend until well combined.

3 Add rice malt syrup and cinnamon, if using, and blend again
until well combined.

4 Pour through a fine-meshed strainer lined with cheesecloth
into a large bowl.

5 Pour coconut milk into a tightly sealed bottle and store in
the fridge for up to a week.

REFERENCES & FURTHER READING

Bueno N et al, 2013. 'Very-low-carbohydrate ketogenic diet v. low-fat diet for long-term weight loss: A meta-analysis of randomised controlled trials', *British Journal of Nutrition*, 110, 7, 178–1187.

Burke LM, 2015. 'Re-examining high-fat diets for sports performance: Did we call the "nail in the coffin" too soon?', *Sports Medicine*, 45 (Suppl 1): 33–49.

Chaix A et al, 2014. 'Time restricted feeding is a preventative and therapeutic intervention against diverse nutritional challenges', *Cell Metabolism*, 20, 6, 991–1005.

Daly ME, 2005. 'Short-term effects of severe dietary carbohydrate-restriction advice in Type 2 diabetes – a randomized controlled trial', *Diabetic Medicine*, 23, 1, 15–20.

De la Monte S and Wands JR, 2008. 'Alzheimer's disease is type 3 diabetes – evidence reviewed', *Journal of Diabetes Science and Technology'*, 2, 6, 1101–1113.

Foster GD et al, 2003. 'A randomized trial of a low-carbohydrate diet for obesity', *New England Journal of Medicine*, 348, 2082–2090.

Fung J and Noakes T, 2016. *The Obesity Code: Unlocking the Secrets of Weight Loss*, Vancouver: Greystone Books.

Kearns CE et al, 2016. 'Sugar industry and coronary heart disease research. A historical analysis of internal industry documents', *Journal of the American Medical Association, Internal Medicine*, 176, 11, 1680–1685.

Lustig R, 2014. *Fat Chance: The Hidden Truth About Sugar, Obesity and Disease*, London: Harper Collins.

McGandy RB et al, 1967. 'Dietary fats, carbohydrates and atherosclerotic vascular disease', *New England Journal of Medicine*, 277, 186–192.

McSwiney FT et al, 2017. 'Keto-adaptation enhances exercise performance and body composition responses to training in endurance athletes', *Metabolism – Clinical and Experimental*, 81, 25–34.

Marinac CR et al, 2015. 'Prolonged nightly fasting and breast cancer risk: Findings from NHANES (2009–2010)', *Cancer Epidemiology, Biomarkers and Prevention*, 24, 783–9.

Marinac CR et al, 2016. 'Prolonged nightly fasting and breast cancer prognosis', *JAMA Oncology*, 2, 8, 1049–1055.

Moore J and Westman E, 2014. *Keto Clarity: Your Definitive Guide to the Benefits of a Low-Carb, High-Fat Diet*, Las Vegas: Victory Belt Publishing Inc.

Phinney SD and Volek J, 2011. *The Art and Science of Low Carbohydrate Living: An Expert Guide to Making the Life-Saving Benefits of Carbohydrate Restriction Sustainable and Enjoyable*, Miami: Beyond Obesity LLC.

Rosch PJ and Harcombe Z, 2016. *Fat and Cholesterol Don't Cause Heart Attacks and Statins Are Not the Solution*, Wales: Columbus Publishing.

Sacks FM et al, 2009. 'Comparison of weight-loss diets with different compositions of fat, protein, and carbohydrates', *New England Journal of Medicine*, 360, 859–873.

Samaha FF et al, 2003. 'A low-carbohydrate as compared with a low-fat diet in severe obesity', *New England Journal of Medicine*, 348, 2074–2081.

Shai I et al, 2008. 'Weight loss with a low-carbohydrate, Mediterranean, or low-fat diet', *New England Journal of Medicine*, 359, 229–241.

Shen R et al, 2016. 'Neuronal energy-sensing pathway promotes energy balance by modulating disease tolerance', *Proceedings of the National Academy of Sciences of the United States of America*, 113, 23, E3307–E3314.

St-Onge M et al, 2017. 'Meal timing and frequency: Implications for cardiovascular disease prevention, A scientific statement from the American Heart Association', *Circulation*, 135 (9), 96–121.

Taubes G, 2006. *The Case Against Sugar*, New York: Alfred A. Knopf.

Taubes G, 2007. *Good Calories, Bad Calories: Challenging the Conventional Wisdom on Diet, Weight Control, and Disease*, New York: Alfred A. Knopf.

Tay J, 2015. 'Comparison of low- and high-carbohydrate diets for type 2 diabetes management: a randomized trial', *American Journal of Clinical Nutrition,* 102, 4, 780–790.

Teicholz N, 2014. *The Big Fat Surprise: Why Butter, Meat and Cheese Belong in a Healthy Diet*, New York: Simon & Schuster.

Volek JS et al, 2009. 'Carbohydrate restriction has a more favorable impact on the metabolic syndrome than a low-fat diet', *Lipids*, 44, 4, 297–309

Volek JS et al, 2016. 'Metabolic characteristics of keto-adapted ultra-endurance runners', *Metabolism – Clinical and Experimental*, 65, 3, 100–110.

Yerushalmy J and Hilleboe HE, 1957. 'Fat in the diet and mortality from heart disease, A methodologic note', *New York State Journal of Medicine*, 57, 2343–54.

Yudkin J and Lustig R, 2016. *Pure, White and Deadly: How Sugar is Killing Us and What We Can Do to Stop It,* London: Penguin Life.

ONLINE RESOURCES

Kombucha: https://thenaturalnutritionist.com.au/learn-how-to-make-your-own-kombucha-with-remedy-kombucha/

Super Easy Bone Broth: https://thenaturalnutritionist.com.au/why-you-shouldnt-be-afraid-of-bone-broth/

Super Easy Kimchi: https://thenaturalnutritionist.com.au/super-easy-kimchi/

ACKNOWLEDGEMENTS

Dr Phil Maffetone, I couldn't have written my first published book and not thank you for your tireless decades of work in our field. Thank you for being the pioneer, for without your work I may have never stumbled across my purpose in life. Your knowledge, your humility and your continuous passion is contagious, and I am honoured to call you a dear friend. Now hurry up and come to Melbourne so I can buy you that coffee!

Peter Brukner, thank you for supporting *Low Carb Healthy Fat Nutrition* and for providing your feedback. It's a dream come true to be collaborating on a topic we are both so passionate about.

Robert Watkins, thank you for your belief in my work and trusting me to deliver this message to Australia and beyond. I am incredibly grateful for the opportunity you have given me, and it's been an absolute pleasure to work together.

Min Benstead, where do I start? They say it takes a village to raise a child, and I say it takes a village to birth a book like this into the world. Thank you for your passion, your creativity and your contribution to The Natural Nutritionist and to this book. I am so proud of you, and to see our recipes come to life like this really is something I am so grateful to share with you.

Sarah Craven, thank you from the bottom of my heart for your creative vision, passion and expertise. You are an absolute dream to work with, and I am honoured to have you wave your magic wand and help to bring my dream to life. Thanks for always knowing my good side and making sure my fringe was in place!

Luke Hines, my friend, you inspire me every day. Thank you for your advice, guidance, support and constant laughs. You really are the funniest person I know and I am so proud to call you one of my closest friends. Thank you for everything you have personally contributed to changing the way the world looks at food. Keep dreaming big, LH!

You, thank you for your support in purchasing this book and continuing to spread the importance of lower carbohydrate, healthy fat nutrition. Your commitment to your health is a big part of why I get to wake up every day and truly live out my dream. Knowledge really is the key to empowerment, and together we can change the world.

INDEX

RECIPE INDEX